Healing
Healthcare

Healing Healthcare

How Doctors and Patients Can Heal Our Sick System

Jeff Kane, MD

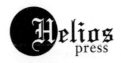

Helios
press

Helios Press books may be purchased in bulk at special discounts for sales promotion, corporate gifts, fund-raising, or educational purposes. Special editions can also be created to specifications. For details, contact the Special Sales Department, Helios Press, 307 West 36th Street, 11th Floor, New York, NY 10018 or info@skyhorsepublishing.com.

19 18 17 16 15   5 4 3 2 1

Published by Helios Press, an imprint of Skyhorse Publishing, Inc.
307 West 36th Street, 11th Floor, New York, NY 10018.

Helios Press® is a registered trademark of Skyhorse Publishing, Inc.®, a Delaware corporation.

www.skyhorsepublishing.com

Cover by Chris Ritchie

Library of Congress Cataloging-in-Publication Data is available on file.

Print ISBN: 978-1-62153-461-7

Ebook ISBN: 978-1-62153-472-3

Printed in the United States of America.

To Veronica Jane Paul,
who's faithfully dragged me,
kicking and screaming,
toward enlightenment

TABLE OF CONTENTS

PREFACE

"The rule books, I'm sure, frown on such intimate engagement
between caregiver and patient. But maybe it's time to rewrite them."

—Kenneth B. Schwartz, Founder,
The Schwartz Center for Compassionate Healthcare

I entered the medical profession a half-century ago, entranced by its celebrated intimacy and altruism. In our secular society, physicianhood was close to a sacred calling. While I practiced, though, I was dismayed to see its aura fade as healthcare deteriorated from a humane service to a relatively impersonal commercial enterprise.

Ironically, that decay resulted from a history of successes. During the twentieth century, scientific medicine—"biomedicine," as we call it—helped us enjoy longer life spans, and wiped out some dread diseases and wrestled others to the mat. Its near-miraculous fruits couldn't help but catch the eye of investors, who encouraged ever more effective, attractive—and profitable—high-tech tests, drugs, and procedures. Popular culture understandably jumped on this promising bandwagon. And that's when healthcare began to turn into a business.

Miracles don't come cheap. It's now common knowledge, for example, that half of recent family bankruptcies were caused by medical expenses. For all its cost, healthcare isn't always worth it. Some of yesterday's "dream drugs" are today's nightmares, and some surgeries first touted as phenomenal now seem a kind of vandalism. Most perniciously, our reliance on medical wizardry has diminished personal responsibility for health.

Of all biomedicine's costs, the most grievous is the loss of what we called "the bedside manner," the doctor's skill of helping sick people feel better simply with his or her own healing presence. Compared to surgical robots and MRI scanners, bedside manner has come to seem relatively wispy, just a little more friendly way of practicing.

We're in the midst of a "healthcare crisis," defined as too little health for far too many bucks. Aching for reform, yet forgetful of the potent centrality of healing presence, we turn to what we can measure, so we understandably conceive healthcare reform simply as a financial challenge.

Happily, bedside manner isn't entirely extinguished. Remnants survive and always will, thanks to a few teachers who preserve the glowing embers. I can no longer recite the catabolic pathway of glycogen, but I remember certain precious educational pearls as though I was handed them yesterday.

Orthopedist Dr. Lorin Stephens, for example, convinced me that medicine wasn't exclusively science's domain. He sat one morning in the mid-1960s with me, three other students, and a psychiatrist, discussing a patient. As the psychiatrist droned Freudian theory, I began to nod off. Noticing that Dr. Stephens was already dozing, the psychiatrist nudged him with his elbow.

"Dr. Stephens," he said, "do you concur?"

Shaking himself awake, Dr. Stephens looked only mildly embarrassed. "Excuse me," he said. "I was dreaming about the smell of my wife's pillow."

Internist Dr. Elsie Giorgi spoke to us about how life situations can result in illness. Realizing we were too inexperienced to appreciate such nuances, she concluded, "All you need to know is this: listen to your patients well enough, and they'll tell you exactly what's going on."

I accompanied Dr. Giorgi to a clinic, where she saw elderly Ms. Grey. Though I was only a junior student, I surmised from Ms. Grey's color and breathing that she had pneumonia. If I'd been her doctor then, I'd have confidently given her antibiotics and moved on to the next patient.

But Dr. Giorgi was deliberately slow. She said, "So, Ms. Grey, tell me about yourself."

The patient said she was raised in a sharecropping family in rural Georgia. She'd married young, suffered two miscarriages, was deserted by her husband, moved, married again and had four children. She'd never had the training or even time to hold a job or escape poverty. She was widowed now, and only two of her children remained alive. Her tale was of lifelong woe. Recently she'd been living with a distant relative who saw to Ms. Grey's upkeep. When the relative died, Ms. Grey, penniless, stopped eating and soon fell ill with pneumonia, which Dr. Giorgi confirmed on examination.

"If we just give Ms. Grey antibiotics," Dr. Giorgi told me, "she'll be back here in two weeks, and then I'll wonder what I'm accomplishing in this business. I'll contact the social worker. Ms. Grey needs someplace to live, and help with nutrition." It had never occurred to me before that a physician's responsibility might transcend the medical setting.

Psychiatry professor Dr. Werner Mendel briefly asked an inpatient small-talk questions before an audience of four medical students. How is it, being on this ward? Is the food okay? How do you spend your day? Then a nurse showed the patient back to the ward, and Dr. Mendel spent the next half-hour delivering a detailed biography of that person, supporting every conclusion with an observation anyone could have made.

"Mr. D's accent places him in a rural area outside New Orleans. He's divorced, judging from the band of pale skin around his left ring finger. The anchor tattoo says he was in the Navy. From his age, I'll say he was in the war, and in the Pacific. Why the Pacific? His little bow when he entered the room—did you see that? [I hadn't]—isn't an American gesture. It's Asian. I'll bet he was in a Japanese POW camp . . ."

Afterward, another psychiatrist read to us from the patient's chart. Dr. Mendel was, as always, astonishingly accurate. Aware of his skill, we students had quaked with vigilance at the edge of our chairs, yet we hadn't absorbed a fraction of the information he'd caught. We hounded him for his secret. All he'd ever say was, "Don't listen to the words. Listen to the music."

The music is the pillow's aroma, the unvoiced story, the symphony emerging from each person's inner universe. When healthcare includes these softer elements, illness exhibits its fuller nature: a misfortune, to be sure, and also a unique narrative rich in meaning and treatment potential.

I'm not the only one to lament the whittling of the medical contact from an intimate encounter down to a bland commercial transaction. Nor am I alone in claiming that simply rearranging healthcare's economics will do little more than postpone its inevitable collapse. And thankfully, I'm only one of thousands who, as you read this, are experimenting with more humane styles of healthcare that, I predict, will revive the bedside manner.

CHAPTER 1

Magic

My mother showed Dr. Gelbard into my room. He sat on my bed and asked me a few questions. Then he felt my burning throat, and it cooled, instantly!

I had no way of knowing he was only checking for enlarged lymph nodes. In my eight-year-old mind, doctors healed by touching. I don't remember the penicillin injection I'm sure he gave me, but I clearly recall that his touch erased my pain. This was magic, and I had to learn it.

A dozen years later, as I applied for entrance to medical school, interviewers asked me the standard question, "Why do you want to be a doctor?"

I was careful not to say, "To learn magic." I gave the preferred response, which was that I loved science and wanted to help people. That was true, too, and good enough.

Orienting us on our first day, the dean listed the classes we'd take: anatomy, physiology, pharmacology, cytology, biochemistry, public health. Something wobbled inside me. Nothing but science? When do I learn how to make people feel better? Maybe they give that course in the second year, or possibly on the wards. Before I was foolish enough to raise my hand and ask the dean, divine providence had me whisper my question to the student beside me.

"Magic?" He screwed up his face. "Did you say 'magic?'"

Ooooo. "Well, er, maybe not exactly, ah, magic, but you know, like, um, bedside manner, whatever. . . ."

"Hey, look, buddy: there's no magic. It's science, period. Get used to it."

I was lucky to have asked him in particular. Today he's a successful psychiatrist.

As he advised, I got used to science and swallowed the traditional oceanic curriculum. As predicted, medicine proved all science and technology. I practiced in a variety of settings, from the National Institutes of Health to county hospital emergency departments, yet my question kept pestering me: where's the magic?

It was there, but below my customary level of perception. Then, thirty years ago, a group of cancer patients who'd taken an information course from the American Cancer Society decided to continue meeting on their own. They invited me to attend, provided I just listened. During my first meeting I realized I was with sick people, yet without the responsibility of being their doctor. Removing my physician filters, I found I could hear their broader stories. I attended the following week and the next, and kept coming. Listening, over months, I learned that sickness, in both its agonies and potential for treatment, is far more than I'd been taught.

Seeking magic, I'd expected to discover something showy— Lazarus raised before my eyes. What I found was invisible, yet undeniably native to healthcare. Personal contact like Dr. Gelbard's touch, mundane and inconspicuous as it is, *alleviates suffering*. It can transform the medical examining room from the utilitarian cubicle it's become back into the sanctuary it was, a healing temple often more potent than drugs or surgery.

Conventional wisdom holds that healthcare reform means financial rearrangement, but in truth, that will barely scratch the surface. Genuine reform will require restoration of the patient-doctor bond, and that will evolve when we question concepts so fundamental we now take them for granted:

- What do we mean by "illness," "treatment," "suffering," "healing," and "cure?"
- What do we mean by "healthcare?"
- How are body and mind related?
- What is a doctor's responsibility? A patient's? A caregiver's?
- What happens when the various participants meet, and what should happen?
- When is it okay to die?
- What level of care do we owe one another?

A national conversation on these issues will guide us toward a more meaningful style of healthcare, one in which:

- We understand that much of illness isn't random, but results from normal aging, socioeconomic disadvantage, and unhealthy habit.
- Physicians consider patients' experiences and perspectives in determining diagnoses and treatments.
- Practitioners address patients' emotional suffering along with their illnesses.
- Caregivers, including professionals, understand they're emotionally affected by their work, and are therefore continually in need of healing themselves.
- Healthcare costs are reduced by relying more on relationships and less on technology.
- We regard healthcare as not just another business, but as profoundly intimate contact, equivalent to a sacrament in religion.

CHAPTER 2

The Healthcare Crisis

I f you've bragged that America enjoys the world's best healthcare, please sit down.

The World Health Organization places the United States in thirty-seventh place for quality, between Costa Rica and Slovenia.

Our sorry rating doesn't result from penny-pinching. On the contrary: we spend 18 percent of our Gross Domestic Product on healthcare while the WHO's number one and two countries, France and Italy, spend less than 12 percent. (That is, one out of every five-and-a-half dollars spent for *anything* in the United States goes toward healthcare; this is triple the proportion we spent in 1960.) According to the International Federation of Health Plans' 2012 report [1] comparing medical prices around the world, a one-day hospital stay in the U.S. costs twenty-six times more than a day in a Spanish hospital. An American appendectomy costs almost eight times more than one done in South Africa. A normal obstetrical delivery in the Netherlands costs a sixth of one in the U.S. (These figures come from those countries' private medical sector, not from their less expensive national medical plans.)

Our costs are so surreally out of line that financial reform is indispensable, but the point of this book is that it can't be the only reform. Breathing new life into the healing relationship will decrease overuse of care by addressing widespread unhealthy life-styles. It will help us avoid romanticizing medical technology. And at long last, it will help us confront our neurotic avoidance of discussing death and dying. Unless we make this change, any conceivable rearrangement of healthcare's finances—whether we remain with the Affordable Care Act ("ACA" or "Obamacare"), adopt a national single-payer plan, or return to our current Byzantine muddle—will drive us toward national bankruptcy without improving our health.

It will help to know how we arrived at today's aggravating jumble. At the turn of the last century, when medical x-rays were experimental and penicillin was only a bread mold, healthcare consisted of the patient, the doctor, and little else.

The leading incurable disease of that pre-antibiotic day was tuberculosis. A prominent specialist, Dr. Edward Livingston Trudeau (1848–1915), developed the first sanitarium shortly after he himself contracted the disease. There, on the shores of Lake Saranac in upstate New York, he offered his patients respite from cities' crowded tenements, along with a serene environment, clean air, and decent food. My own aunt's two years at Trudeau's establishment granted her another seven decades of life. The sanitarium is now a research facility. Beneath the vines obscuring Trudeau's statue, a brass plaque commemorates his motto:

"Cure sometimes,
Relieve often,
Comfort always."

Dr. Trudeau was a steward of an ancient tradition. In medieval Europe, before there were hospitals as we know them, churches like Paris' ancient Hôtel Dieu took in the sick. Its nuns dispensed the medicines of the time, most of which ranged from useless to toxic. When patients improved, then, it wasn't from medications as much as from inhabiting a sacred place, being bathed in stained glass light, and given food, rest, quiet, kindness, hope, and dignity.

Dr. Trudeau's style contrasted with that of contemporaries who practiced solely via drugs and physical interventions. Psychologist Lawrence LeShan compared the two approaches in his 1982 book, *The Mechanic and the Gardener*. When something breaks, a mechanic learns how it works in order to repair it, while a gardener nurtures and supports, trusting that healing, if it's to happen, results naturally.

The late Victorian era was the Golden Age of the Mechanic. Industrial barons John D. Rockefeller and Andrew Carnegie found it absurd that while Americans were driving Henry Ford's new automobiles, their healthcare lurched about in a virtual horse-and-buggy. The enterprises calling themselves medical schools ranged from universities to carnival booths. The Illinois Board of Health reported in 1899 that one hundred seventy-nine American and Canadian medical schools featured some degree of scientific approach, twenty-six taught homeopathy (unscientific, according to the Board), another twenty-six were "eclectic," thirteen "miscellaneous," and thirteen were outright frauds. Carnegie and Rockefeller jointly resolved to replace this jumble with a standardized system suited to modern times. E. Richard Brown, late UCLA professor of health policy, tells the fascinating story in his book *Rockefeller Medicine Men*.

Rockefeller assigned reform to his administrator of philanthropies, the Rev. Frederick T. Gates. A citizen of his mechanical times, Gates viewed the human body as a physical plant vulnerable to disease's criminal assault. He wrote to Rockefeller,

> "The body has a network of insulated nerves, like telephone wires, which transmit instantaneous alarms at every point of danger. The body is furnished with a most elaborate police system, with hundreds of police stations to which the criminal elements are carried by the police and jailed. . . . The body has a most complete and elaborate sewer system . . ."

Feeling strongly that science should be the exclusive basis of medical education, Gates founded the Rockefeller Institute for Medical Research (now Rockefeller University) in 1901. Though he encountered little direct opposition, a few instructors expressed polite misgivings. One was Dr. William Osler, professor of medicine at Johns Hopkins University, regarded even today as the patriarch of North American medicine. Though he revered science, Osler insisted throughout his career that human beings couldn't be healed by science alone. He called his own practice style a necessary composite of science and art, or, as LeShan would later put it, mechanics plus gardening. Said Osler,

> "The practice of medicine is an art, not a trade; a calling, not a business; a calling in which your heart will be exercised equally with your head. Often the best part of your work will have nothing to do with powders or potions . . ."

Here's a typical story of Osler as gardener, related by medical philosophy author Dr. Larry Dossey in the foreword he wrote for my book *How To Heal*:

Dr. Osler headed one morning to a graduation ceremony in his full academic regalia—robe, hood, sashes, medals. On the way, he visited the home of his friend and colleague, Ernest Mallam. Mallam's son was sick with whooping cough and appeared to be dying. He didn't respond to the ministrations of his parents or the nurses, but when Osler appeared in his sartorial grandery, the boy was captivated. After a brief examination, Osler peeled a peach, cut and sugared it, and fed it bit by bit to the enthralled boy. Although he felt recovery was unlikely, he returned daily for the next forty days, each time dressed in his robes, and personally fed the child, who ultimately did recover.

Osler was disappointed that his warnings about science eclipsing art were all but ignored by Rockefeller, Carnegie, and Gates. He left Johns Hopkins in 1904 for Oxford University, writing to a colleague he considered too laboratory-oriented, "Now I go, and you have your way."

To generate support for scientizing medical education, Carnegie commissioned educator Abraham Flexner to critically examine its current state. Competent and thorough, Flexner visited every medical school in the country. In his final report, issued in 1910, he recommended that curricula and methods be uniform and based on science.

Medical students since then have learned during their first week that the Flexner Report marked the historical boundary between healthcare as a Victorian relic and as modern biomedicine. Contributing over a hundred million dollars, Carnegie and Rockefeller established facilities and science-based teaching chairs at America's major medical schools. Unfunded institutions soon found competition difficult, and in a few years half of America's medical schools closed.

This isn't ancient history. Science's domination of medical education occurred only yesterday: my own instructors received their training from students of the professors Carnegie and Rockefeller funded.

Never would those philanthropists have dreamed the magnitude of their ensuing success. Over the next century their efforts would make possible organ transplants, gene recoding, polio immunizations, and numerous other advances. They'd be chagrined, though, to learn that biomedicine's achievements would ironically create its obsolescence.

CHAPTER 3

The Fall of Biomedicine

B iomedicine's successes were so spectacular that the limelight deservedly shined on "mechanics" while "gardeners" receded into the shadows . . . that is, until recently, since for all that biomedicine's achieved, it now bumps up against the ceiling Dr. Osler predicted. [1]

Its most obvious limit is its inexhaustible cost. As healthcare technology increasingly flourished, fewer patients carried enough cash to pay up-front, so various financial innovations attempted to ease the expense. The precursor to Blue Cross was founded in 1929 by a group of Dallas teachers who contracted with Baylor University Hospital to provide twenty-one days of hospitalization for a fixed six-dollar payment.

Not bad, but it's grown. Last year my sixty-year-old friend Mike had the cheapest California Blue Shield policy, costing $5,100 annually. (Some might claim this was insurance in name only, since it required an annual $5,200 deductible and $5,200 co-pay.)

As I write this, Mike is exploring the Affordable Care Act's website to locate a new policy, which he hopes, as the program's name suggests, will be affordable. It'll likely carry a deductible, and once Mike has met that, the insurance carrier, Blue Shield or some other, will begin to pay his medical bills. At that point the company, not Mike, will become the doctor's employer. Subsequent decisions involving his care will no longer be an issue solely between him and his doctor. Their relationship will be impacted, if not wholly directed, by the interests of an entity that knows neither of them and views healthcare exclusively in measurable, that is, mechanical terms.

Another of biomedicine's limits resulted ironically from its stupendous achievements. Along with public health interventions, it extended American life expectancy from fifty-two years at the time of Flexner's report to seventy-eight today. The 2010 U.S. census revealed that the median age in America reached its highest point ever that year: 37.2 years, up from 35.3 years in 2000 and 32.9 years in 1990.

More people are living to an age at which they encounter a different kind of illness than they would have when young. The child biomedicine helped to survive diphtheria in 1945 is now a senior, subject to the obstinate effects of aging. One afternoon, as I listened to some members of our cancer support group lament their arthritis pains, constipation woes, and dental troubles, I realized that survival had delivered them to old age, with its own array of infirmities.

Seniors just look elderly to the young, but when it's you who occupies those wrinkles, much of your day reminds you that you're wearing out. Medical science can extend life expectancy, but it will never eliminate aging, which is why a poll would no doubt show that older people aren't as interested in extending their sojourn as younger ones are. I'd love to live with a sharp mind and unblemished skin forever, but these days that prospect is as likely as a shrimp singing an aria. I try to picture myself at a hundred and fifty, spiking volleyballs on a tropical sugar beach and then retiring to a sex-drenched siesta, but what I see instead is my desiccated form in the sand, barely distinguishable from driftwood.

Let's face it: aging is slow decomposition. Hardly anything—the immune system, reflexes, memory, sphincters, charm, you name it—functions as well as it once did. Days fly by ever more rapidly, and so do our organs, hopefully in single file rather than *en masse*. Medical treatment will smooth some of aging's discomforts and buy some time, but there will be no cure. Aging isn't one of God's mistakes; it's *normal*.

Indefinite life extension is a fool's errand anyway. Exploring immortality's social consequences, Kurt Vonnegut wrote a story in which seventeen generations had to crowd into single apartments. People died, usually from defenestration. Look it up.

We can't cure aging, but if we get used to it, we might find an occasional gem in the gravel. For example, we seniors can find pleasure in our hormones no longer whipping us around. Or maybe someone appreciates us for the few grains of wisdom we've gleaned from longevity. When I hit the hundred mark and journalists dutifully ask my secret, I hope I can omit the bit about daily cigars and Jack Daniels, and say instead that I simply wanted to be around longer because I'd crafted such a good life from what I'd been given.

The hurting elderly need their physical symptoms treated, and they also need alleviation of their emotional suffering along with guidance in living more gracefully with maturity's toll. No mechanic can help here; this is a gardener's task. Dr. Trudeau would have accepted this challenge, but his successors in biomedicine aren't tooled for it.

Twentieth-century biomedicine's glamorous prowess stole the stage from more subtle low-tech intimacy. The laboratory replaced the sanctuary. House calls disappeared as doctors' little black bags couldn't accommodate x-ray machines and electrolyte analyzers.

In fact, medical machinery became so effective, pervasive, and persuasive that we came to equate it with healthcare itself. Several years ago, a television crew interviewed me about cancer support groups. Meetings consist purely of conversation; our most complex tool is Kleenex. Was the story introduced on the air with a graphic of two people talking? No, a stethoscope. Absent scientific apparatus, how would the audience recognize that the story was about healthcare?

Now, when we think of the "bedside manner" at all, it's as fuzzy pleasantness rather than the chief tool for alleviating suffering. Depending on the relative presence or absence of authentic bedside manner, the patient will see the physician as either a healer or a clocked-in technician.

A deficient patient-doctor relationship is the origin of most liability litigation. For years our hospital's attorneys gave the medical staff a periodic talk about how to avoid malpractice suits. Their message was always, "Most suits arise not from damage, even when real damage has occurred. People sue when they're angry. And they're least angry at—and most likely to forgive—physicians who care about them. So to stay out of court, develop a close relationship with your patients."

That advice resonates with the Hippocratic Oath's directive to put patients' welfare first. But physicians too discover that the Oath conflicts with rules and regulations of the government agencies, insurance corporations, and accountants who are their employers. Any doctor will be happy to tell you of some recent time he or she felt that frustrating conflict.

A close relationship is a trusting one. When I know and have faith in my doctor, I'll accept his or her clinical assessment of me. When we've only just met, though, I might ask for a further test, just to be on the safe side. And if I'm that doctor, I, too, might ask for that extra test, just to be on the safe side. That is, the closer the relationship, all else equal, the less it's likely to cost.

Note that I'm criticizing current healthcare's inordinate reliance on technology, not technology itself. Nor do patients have anything against technology. When I hear occasional complaints from them about their care, it's never about medicine's high-tech tools. Instead, they uniformly lament deficiencies in healthcare's lowest-tech aspect, communication. Too often, patients say, they're treated almost like bystanders.

A convalescing friend told me, "When I was in the hospital, I was poked and probed and *ultraviolated*, but never touched." Others have said:

"My doctor doesn't face me. He just types into his laptop."

"I waited all day by the phone for the call the clinic promised. Never came."

"When I was hospitalized, the only staff member who just sat down and talked with me was the janitor."

"No one asked me whether I could afford this prescription, eighty bucks a pill."

"It feels like my doctor always keeps one hand on the doorknob."

"I hear about the importance of diet, exercise, and coping with stress, but no doctor's ever asked me a thing about how I live my life."

"How is it medical science can transplant half our organs, but can't fax my test results across town?"

These examples may seem minor annoyances, but patients can conclude from their prevalence that medical people often practice hardly knowing, let alone comforting them.

The fading of the patient-doctor relationship means each participant is less visible to the other. Indeed, they've each been conceptually reduced. The way we as patients see ourselves— our tastes, values, hopes, and skills, our individualities—isn't as important, in the biomedical view, as our organs, tissues, and cells. See one patient unit, you've seen them all. Little notice is taken of personal contributions to our illnesses or to the resources we might bring to our own care. And physicians, as interchangeable "providers," likewise suffer discounting of their unique attributes.

Recalling Dr. Trudeau (p. 5) and Dr. Osler (p. 7), I see an image of patient and doctor sitting knee-to-knee and heart-to-heart. As a matter of fact, that looks today as quaint as a Norman Rockwell painting . . . and exactly what we need.

CHAPTER 4

Not Your Parents' Illnesses

Illness isn't what it used to be. Its prime cause has shifted from germs to, well, *us*. A staggering number of us live unhealthily. Ask your doctor what proportion of his or her patients endure some combination of detrimental diet, inadequate exercise, toxic exposure, adverse self-image, poor stress management, unfulfilling work, deficient support, and dysfunctional relationships. When I ask my colleagues, they uniformly answer three-quarters and upward. We docs call such behaviors "pathogenic," or sick-making, as they'll bloom into obesity, diabetes, hypertension, atherosclerosis, emphysema, and a horde of other maladies, most of which will prove as chronic and intractable as those of aging.

"Chronic," by the way, means long-term. Before 1960, two-thirds of medical visits were for "acute," or short-termed, conditions. Principally infections and trauma, they either went their way or carried you off after a few days or weeks. Biomedicine is particularly well-equipped to address acute disorders. After 1960, though, the ratio began to reverse, largely due to biomedicine's success, and today two-thirds of medical visits are for chronic conditions. They're lengthy only because they're incurable. In fact, *"chronic" is a euphemism for "incurable."* We'd cure your arthritis or ALS or lupus if we could, but we can't, so you'll have it a long time, probably the rest of your life.

Chronicity, including the trials of aging and the obstinate results of pathogenic behavior, is now healthcare's dominant challenge. For most patients, biomedicine—the application of complex, sometimes invasive, hazardous, and always costly technologies—amounts to shooting golden bullets at mirage targets. We routinely intervene too late, when the damage has been done; while we expensively repair the barn door, the horse is already three pastures away. However impressive our science, it too often disappoints our patient. Biomedicine is useful in reducing the symptoms of chronic disorders, but what will help at least as much is the addition of skillful comforting and counseling. That's a crucial intervention, since what we actually suffer from isn't our diagnoses as much as our emotional reactions to them.

A perfect example is cancer, largely a disease of older people, and which for most patients becomes a chronic illness. Many cancers, especially in early stages, display no symptoms at all. The majority of prostate, colon, and cervical cancers are silent for months to years. We feel well when we visit the doctor—that is, until he or she uses the "C" word. The moment we hear that, our lives shred into confetti. It feels like we've been abducted and abandoned in *terra incognita*. When newly diagnosed people attend our support group for the first time, they're commonly distressed beyond speech. Their cancer status before and after diagnosis hasn't changed, so it's not their tumors terrorizing them. It's their own normal—and treatable—emotional response to the news.

Cancer, congestive heart failure, Parkinsonism, autoimmune diseases, and other chronic processes don't simply hang around our home like trash in the garage. They move into the living room, permanently, and then snoop around to enlarge their quarters. With these troublesome new residents occupying our home and no eviction forthcoming, we realize we need more than physical help; we need patience, tolerance, strength, and assertiveness as well.

Before arthritis affected you, you opened jars without a thought, and now all you can do is strain, grunt, and finally ask for help—and this is just one of your limitations. Or you feel your social life crumble as your cancer and its treatment leave you unable to plan even for tomorrow. You begin to feel diminished, dependent, and even helpless in some areas of your life. Over years, this slowly slides toward depression. But arthritis or cancer is the culprit only indirectly; what's more responsible for getting you down is your response to it, your normal emotions.

Biomedical doctors laudably attempt to slow your illness' progression and diminish your pain with their "armamentarium," as they call it. When more intense symptoms appear, they offer you more serious drugs or more invasive surgery. You eventually find yourself at a difficult crossroad, pondering whether to opt for ever more drastic treatments or just accept your symptoms and go home and enjoy a hot cup of tea.

Biomedicine's committed focus on illness' physical aspect devalues if not ignores the patient's experience. For example, a *TIME* magazine cover photo a few years ago depicted an eleven-year-old girl with type two diabetes, a disease that until then had been the bane of the obese middle-aged, and unheard of in children. But now, according to the story, kids were regularly contracting it. The article mentioned, almost in passing, that this girl weighed two-hundred-twenty pounds.

Hold on, I thought, wait a minute. How does an eleven-year-old come to weigh two-hundred-twenty pounds? How much sugar and processed foods are in her diet? And how is it that her weight is only a sidebar, not the story's center? What have her parents done about it? Why isn't this child's history as important as her disease? Reading and re-reading the piece, I found nothing further about her, but scads about insulin metabolism, surgical procedures, and new drugs on the way.

Here's why we can no longer ignore a two-hundred-twenty-pound eleven-year-old's life: a half-century ago, our principal foe was germs, but today much of our own behavior spawns illness.

The most prominent "pathogenic" (disease-making) style is eating too much of the wrong stuff, so I'll focus on that first.

According to the U.S. Centers for Disease Control and Prevention, a third of American adults are obese. "Overweight" and "obese" are technical terms. If you'd like to know where you fit in, divide your weight in pounds by the square of your height in inches, and multiply the result by 703. For example, if you weigh 140 pounds and are five feet six inches (that is, sixty-six inches) tall, your calculation would be

$$\frac{140}{66 \times 66} \times 703 = 22.59$$

The result, here 22.59, is your "body mass index," or BMI. If your BMI is between twenty-five and thirty, you're overweight, and above thirty, obese.

Obesity is getting to be the American way. A new hospital wing I visited features a dedicated obesity ward fitted with a hydraulic lift system, as its employees, many of whom are overweight themselves, are at physical risk raising and moving thousands of pounds of patients daily. A man recently sued a fast-food chain because its seats wedged him in too tightly. Some clothing companies have reset their "normal," relabeling large-size clothes as more petite to persuade customers that they still fit into smaller garments.

The airlines, where too heavy a payload can be lethal, have adjusted their norms, too. In 2005, the FAA updated average passenger weights used in calculating each flight's mass and balance. Men's weight was raised by twenty-five pounds, to two hundred, and women's by thirty-four pounds, to one hundred seventy-nine. (Those are the summer figures, when passengers dress lightly; the winter figures are higher.)

When as a child I asked my mother why some people were obese, she replied, "Glands." That was the assumption *du jour*.

Today's assumptions include familial practices, inactivity, pharmaceutical effects, and always-popular genetics (almost daily we hear about the discovery of a gene that "predisposes" its host toward obesity or addiction or, I predict, loyalty to the Chicago Cubs).

Maybe each of those factors exerts some influence, but none compare to the sweet toxicity of the American diet: we eat a literally sickening amount of sugar. Eighty percent of food items in American supermarkets contain added sugar. If you don't believe me, cruise the aisles reading labels; by the way, sugar is often disguised with dozens of other names, my favorite being "evaporated cane juice".[1] For an adult of normal body mass index (BMI), the World Health Organization recommends no more than twenty-five grams—six teaspoons—of sugar daily. Compare that with a single twelve-ounce Coca-Cola, which contains thirty-nine grams of sugar. People commonly drink more than one.

When we ingest sugar, the pancreas secretes insulin, which directs cells to absorb it for fuel. Excess sugar is stored as fat. I know a man who drinks ten cans of Mountain Dew daily; that amounts to more than a pound of sugar, or about eighteen times the WHO allowance every day. If he keeps it up, eventually his insulin will lose effectiveness ("insulin resistance"), resulting in the high levels of blood sugar and insulin we call type two diabetes. It's predicted that, at current rates of impairment, 95 percent of Americans will be overweight or obese in two decades, and by 2050, one out of every three Americans will be diabetic.

Diabetes isn't like nearsightedness, which can be corrected with glasses. Even when medicated, it's a major risk factor for heart and blood vessel disease and damage to the eyes, nerves, kidneys, and extremities.

Sugar's ubiquity is a particularly serious problem for poorer people in neighborhoods of limited real-food availability. If you're living on little, you'll likely eat processed foods notoriously richer in sugar and chemicals than in sustenance. Plump but unnourished, unfit, easily fatigued, and with compromised immunity, you, who can afford healthcare least, will suffer a gaggle of medical disorders.

Sugar's our main obesity source, but not the only one. Some of us are overweight because we simply eat too much. We usually can't say why, but sometimes clues emerge in our language. One portly man, indicating the immense food warehouse in which he worked, told me, "I'm into food storage." Another man giggled, "I'm such an airhead that if I didn't carry all this ballast I'd just float away." A woman told me others made her uncomfortable, and her extra weight served as a kind of emotional buffer. Others express variants of a particular theme, an attempt to fill what's empty. A country song now making the rounds goes like this:

> I bought me an RV to travel,
> and seek what might comfort my soul,
> To see if I was more than a food tube,
> an unfillable, bottomless hole.
> I parked in the lot of a Walmart
> and in high hopes I entered the store.
> I bought an iPod and a drill
> and a George Foreman grill,
> But left as empty as I was before.

Geneen Roth, author of *When Food Is Love* and other books on eating disorders, advises, "You can't get enough of what you don't need." Millions of us acquire iPods, drills, and George Foreman grills in an unconscious attempt to fill an existential void, to remedy the sensation that we're excruciatingly empty, devoid of purpose. This isn't a physical disorder, but a spiritual one, so no amount of food, consumer goods, medicines, or surgeries will fix it any more than we can splint a broken promise.

If we were sufficiently alarmed about morphing into an obese, sickly America (with even higher healthcare costs), we'd develop a crash strategy equivalent to the Manhattan Project. We'd generate nationwide educational programs, town hall meetings, door-to-door volunteer contacts, parenting circles, youth fitness clubs, you name it.

But attempts regularly meet resistance. Consider the New York City ordinance, introduced by mayor Michael Bloomberg in 2012 (and judicially voided a year later) that banned soft drink servings larger than sixteen ounces. Opponents raised a slew of objections, largely along the lines of meddling "nanny" government. The NAACP and the Hispanic Federation charged that the soda rule would unduly harm minority businesses and reduce freedom of choice in low-income communities. (Perhaps not coincidentally, those two groups have received grants or sponsorship funds from Coca-Cola and PepsiCo.)[2]

I assumed Bloomberg put forth his ordinance to publicize the hazards of massive soft drink ingestion. I'd like to believe some citizens took him seriously and stopped buying these products. In any case, the rule was only advisory, since anyone could finish a sixteen-ounce Coke and buy a second one.

Another strategy is biomedicine's, which, true to its character, is to put obese kids on drugs. A report issued in 2011 by the National Heart, Lung, and Blood Institute (NHLBI) advocated checking children age nine and up for serum cholesterol, and medicating those with high fat levels. (The report also mentioned deploying "intense lifestyle management," but didn't say what that might consist of; in fact, there's been so little development of effective behavioral interventions that the approach will essentially be drugs.) Soon American children might take medications not only for their attention deficit disorder, but for their high cholesterol, too. Then again, maybe this plan isn't so surprising when we learn that half the authors of the NHLBI report have had drug industry ties.

Obesity is only one form of sick-making behavior. Twenty percent of us still smoke cigarettes. Of Americans who have even heard of stress management, precious few practice it. We drink too much alcohol, exercise reluctantly, take more drugs than we need, rush through "meals" of fake food, paddle a virtual sea of environmental toxins, put up with superficial or even dreadful relationships, and lustily accept frenzied consumerism, driving to work and working to drive, with a cell phone in one hand and a McGutbuster in the other.

Why don't we more urgently address the noxious elements in our food, air, and water? Mainly because we misunderstand how poisons work. In our fast-paced society, instant action registers more readily than a slowly unfolding event, so we conceive of poisoning as Socrates drinking hemlock and falling over dead. Yet I can down ten Mountain Dews a day and remain standing, so what gives?

The results of most poisons, including sugar, don't appear instantly, but build gradually as effects accumulate over long periods. Light up a cigarette and you won't crumple today, but smoke thirty pack-years, and your lungs will reliably turn to nonfunctional lace. The equivalent is true for many carcinogens, heavy metals . . . and American quantities of sugar.

It's not as if we don't know better. We've been encouraged as long as I can remember to brush and floss, eat sensibly, exercise, and learn to address stress. Cigarettes are now so heavily taxed and carry warnings so lurid that only the most determined smokers purchase them.

What can possibly motivate unhealthy, self-thwarting behavior? One tantalizing suspect is low self-esteem. A tattered self-image arguably drives much of depression, eating disorders, accident-proneness, hostility, social withdrawal, underachievement, and, ironically, overachievement (CEOs, politicians, and celebrities, take note). If we didn't believe we somehow deserve it, why

would we allow ourselves and our children to marinate in the toxins that permeate the biosphere? A people who felt more worthy
would be at the barricades, waving pikes and clubs.

Low self-esteem can confine us to social circles in which
we're unseen, unheard, untouched, and unappreciated. (People
speak about wretched relationships these days with an openness
that suggests dysfunction is the norm. I saw a cartoon showing a
half-dozen people scattered around a huge auditorium under the
banner, "Annual Conference of Functional Families.") Assuming
it's us at fault, we stuff our consequent despair. Beneath that happy
face can gurgle a swamp of unwholesome concepts, including:

- There's something basically wrong with me
- If I revealed more of who I really am, no one would
  like me
- I have little to offer the world
- I am how I am, and can't change
- I need someone else to tell me what I should do
- I can't change anything, so why bother?
- If I ignore it, it'll go away

Much of psychotherapy, when all's said and done, amounts to
the client accepting, finally, that he or she is okay. It just takes
awhile for that to penetrate the defensive rationalizations. You probably know someone who tolerates a loveless marriage, unrewarding
career, and shallow friendships, but who, if asked, "How are you
doing?" would answer, "Terrific!" Yet actions speak louder than
words. The truth inevitably emerges from the body, sometimes as
illness. Poet-visionary William Blake wasn't just gibbering when he
advised, "He who desires but acts not breeds pestilence."

Enhanced self-esteem might prod us to question whether nominal public guardians are really looking out for us. For example, the Food and Drug Administration maintains a large list of industrial and commercial chemicals it defines as "GRAS," Generally Recognized As Safe. These substances, found in everything from insecticides to children's cereals, remain untested despite the well-known principle that biohazards can take decades or whole generations to manifest. In addition, it's hard to discern the precise action of one type of molecule among—and in concert with—hundreds or thousands of others.

It may surprise you to know that America affords chemicals the same status as criminal defendants—innocent until proven guilty beyond a reasonable doubt. Consider Canada's contrasting approach to this issue. Under its "precautionary principle," chemicals are banned unless there's scientific consensus that they're long-term safe.

If we were proactive, we could prevent most cancers. In his Pulitzer Prize–winning book *The Emperor of All Maladies*, oncologist Siddhartha Mukherjee emphasizes repeatedly that the most effective and safest treatment for cancer isn't chemo, radiation, or surgery. It's prevention. I'm not talking about reversing some "cancer personality," as some people suggest, but ridding our environment of its resident carcinogens.

Of course, powerful economic interests are happy to encourage inertia in these matters. Energy companies would rather we didn't know what chemicals are in the high-pressure slurry used to fracture ("frack") underground faults (and which mix with potable aquifers) to extract natural gas. Plastic manufacturers resist attempts to ban bisphenol A (BPA) from drink containers and food cans. Monsanto, Dow, and their corporate cousins invested millions to defeat Proposition 37 in

California, which would have mandated labeling (not banning, just labeling) genetically modified foods.

Taken together, pathogenic behaviors, including civic paralysis, can look like enactment of a not-so-subtle death wish. But that's hardly ever the case. On the contrary, it's usually a grab at life, an attempt to cope with social demands. Young adults who begin to smoke do so not to wreck their lungs, but because their friends smoke, encouraged by cigarette ads touting that sought-after *savoir-faire* image. Alcoholics don't drink to bring on cirrhosis, but to anesthetize the pain in their life. A teenager doesn't escape into the video game world aiming to stunt his maturation, but to play a game he can win. The compulsive consumer, unconsciously shopping for spiritual fulfillment, settles for a hot fudge sundae or new shoes. The employee or spouse who puts up with abuse does so because the prospect of responding honestly is scarier than simply going along to get along. Citizens who avert their eyes from environmental vandalism aren't evil corporate agents, just people trying to get by in these tough times.

If, as I suggest, unhealthy behavior's intent is survival rather than self-destruction, then much of illness' origin is social—choices attempting to accommodate to society's unhealthy values. Unfortunately, sociology is an area outside biomedical jurisdiction. Untrained as public health agents or psychotherapists who might prevent illness by influencing behavior, we doctors can only wait for patients to show up for repairs after their organs cave in. The source of their behavior—their consciousness, values, and emotions—isn't our responsibility since it's not scientifically addressable, being intangible, invisible, and unmeasurable. To biomedicine, these fundamental human functions are literally and figuratively immaterial, a word that also means irrelevant.

CHAPTER 5

The Healthcare Industry

"In the United States today, we give you all the care you can afford, whether or not you need it, as opposed to all the care you need, whether or not you can afford it."

—Dr. Arthur Kellermann, Former Associate Dean
Emory University School of Medicine

During the past fifty years, biomedicine's ever-more-expensive gear was a flashing beacon to the profit-minded. They climbed aboard and restructured healthcare, year by year, from a human service into an industry. Now it's so firmly commercial that people under forty scarcely know it was ever otherwise. Today healthcare is considered a commodity like oil or pork bellies, a standardized product to be taken from its shelf by a "provider," a doctor, and sold to a patient, a "consumer."

During the same recent period, we've witnessed a huge rise in lifestyle-generated illnesses along with an increasingly older population, but haven't adjusted medical practice accordingly. We could have demanded less reliance on mechanics and more attention to gardening, particularly education and counseling, but the fact is that there's more money in machinery.

Business' sway over healthcare can't be overstated. Beneath its banner, commercially unadaptable elements predictably wilt. Stanford University researcher Dr. David Spiegel was lead author of a 1989 study indicating that women with breast cancer who participated in support groups enjoyed twice the survival time of women not in groups. (Though subsequent studies contested this conclusion, it was bombshell news upon its publication in the prestigious journal *Lancet*.) Responding to the medical orthodoxy's surprisingly paltry interest in his work, Spiegel said, "If my intervention was a new chemotherapy agent, every hospital in the country would be doing it by now. But it wasn't a drug. It was simply conversation. Who's going to promote that, chair manufacturers?"

As healthcare morphed into retail trade, the patient and physician had to make space in the safe haven of their examining room for insurance clerks, government bureaucrats, drug company reps, technology marketers, and attorneys, not to mention the ever-proliferating hardware. Today the room's so crowded that the original occupants can barely hear one another.

Physician demographics have followed the economic trend. Least-specialized family practice ("primary care") offers a doctor the widest view of the patient . . . and the lowest income. According to one study, median income for family docs was $162,000 in 2004, the least of any practice, while specialists earned a median $297,000, with cardiologists and radiologists exceeding $400,000.

This is a serious difference when you're entering practice with hundreds of thousands in education debt. Never trained in business, you're suddenly over your ears in red ink. Little wonder that the proportion of medical school graduates entering family practice has consistently dropped over the past decade. Instead they swell specialties, in which physical procedures pay handsomely. A dermatologist removing a mole earns more in fifteen minutes than a family doc who counsels a patient for an hour.

Not that a mole shouldn't be removed, or that some other procedure shouldn't be performed. Medical technology can be truly wondrous. Yet the decision to employ it is too often motivated by business factors rather than medical considerations, such as the blandishments of pharmaceutical salespeople, or the need to amortize equipment. In fact, healthcare has become so inextricable from business that one can hardly address any of its aspects—doctors' attitudes, diagnosis, testing, liability, treatments—without reference to economics.

To maintain my license, I attended continuing medical education luncheons. The hosts, Avarice Pharmaceuticals or one of its cousins, attracted maximum attendance with delectable cuisine. While we docs savored our *crème brûlée*, the speaker, a prestigious psychiatry professor, informed us that we'd been grossly under-diagnosing clinical depression. Were we to perform properly, we'd have more patients on Avarice's best-seller, Happyzac™.

This looked to me like barefaced bribery, but the colleagues I asked considered it plain old education. One told me, "Don't be so cynical. It's fair, after all: every company has its opportunity. Last month we heard from Drugs-R-Us about Ecstasoft™, didn't we?"

Over years, such presentations, albeit hosted by competing companies, relentlessly reinforce the notion that whether we use this drug or that drug, drugs are the answer. Non-drug approaches like counseling or dietary education are valuable, but they never dished up *crevettes étouffées*. In addition to its free-lunch infomercials and doctor-lobbying, the industry runs full-page magazine ads encouraging readers to ask their doctor for the pill—or the test or surgical procedure—that will fix their lives.

A massive industry encouraging patients to demand more medical care is a major reason healthcare is so expensive. The usual suspects—medical fees, hospital billing practices, malpractice issues—aren't the villains, only consequences of our mesmerization by biomedicine's promises.

For example, *every day* in 2008, almost five hundred patients underwent hundred-thousand-dollar-plus coronary artery bypass operations in the United States. Most of these procedures are of an urgent nature, and at that point must be done. But how much attention do we direct toward earlier intervention, before the situation becomes dire? Solid research [1] shows that a program of diet, exercise, support, and meditation delivers benefits at least equal to those of surgery, and at about 4 percent of the cost, but it's most effective when initiated before cardiac symptoms appear.

Another example of our indoctrinated default toward technology can be found in the *AARP News*, which, after periodically cautioning against excessive healthcare usage, suggested in its June 2011 issue that obese readers look into gastric bypass surgery at forty thousand dollars a pop.

One rewarding marketing strategy is to "medicalize" a facet of normal life, change a common function into a treatable diagnosis. Psychiatry's bible, the Diagnostic and Statistical Manual of Mental Disorders (DSM), was recently revised into a fifth edition. The previous version had excluded bereavement as a diagnosis, since sadness after loss is normal. But since bereavement can descend into clinical depression, some therapists insisted on formally monitoring it by retaining it in the book. Opponents claimed this would medicalize normal bereavement, exposing sufferers to drug-oriented practitioners. The "DSM-5 Task Force" finally decided to include it as a diagnosis. So if you're currently grieving, you might be ripe for Avarice Pharmaceuticals' blockbuster drug, NoGriefia™.

How do such rules come into being? I looked up the bios of the twenty-nine DSM-5 task force members.[2] I stopped after perusing the first eleven, since I have a life to live. Of that number, nine reported associations with pharmaceutical companies, either as consultant, stockholder, or grant or honorarium recipient.

According to a report prepared by the U.S. Centers for Disease Control and Prevention,[3] more than ten thousand American toddlers two to three years old are being medicated for attention

deficit hyperactivity disorder (ADHD). The report found that toddlers covered by Medicaid—that is, from poorer families—are
particularly prone to be put on medications such as Ritalin and
Adderall.

The treatment is beyond questionable, since the American
Academy of Pediatrics doesn't recognize ADHD in children three
years and younger, let alone approve the use of drugs to treat it.
Giving toddlers such potent drugs looks so risky on its face that one
wonders why docs would recommend it. One easy answer is that
patients don't like to leave doctors' offices without some talisman—a
drug sample, appointment slip, prescription—signifying they were
seen and ostensibly helped. A thorough consultation would usually
be of more use, but that won't earn the practice a cent, and scrawling
a prescription accelerates the patient flow.

Where does such an ill-advised practice come from?
Unsupported within conventional medicine, it must have arisen
elsewhere; my guess is that drug reps recommend it to docs as
"off-label."

Off-label prescribing means the doc has decided the drug, though
not indicated, is worth a try. In medicalese this is called an "empiri-
cal" trial, not "a toss of the dice." If it seems to work, no one will care
about its propriety. Off-label prescribing is surprisingly common.
According to a report in *Health Affairs*,[4] 21 percent of prescriptions for one hundred sixty common drugs in the United States were
for off-label indications. Of these prescriptions, one hundred fifty
million of them, 73 percent, had little or no scientific support.

When I practiced standard medicine I, like most docs, was visited
by pharmaceutical representatives. They were uniformly friendly,
good-looking, well-dressed, personable, and dreadfully smart. When
they educated me about their products, including off-label uses, I
knew they were cooing the best features and withholding the worst.
But I was too busy at the time to learn what they *didn't* tell me.

If I sold pharmaceuticals, I'd be an idiot to begin my ads with the drug's six hundred possible side effects. I'd craft a more attractive introduction, maybe the image of the world's best-looking sexagenarian, ecstatic after sinking a hole-in-one. I'd place the list of side effects on the next page, in three-point migraine type.

Maybe that's fair, business being business, after all. But it doesn't stop there. Corners get cut until there's hardly much truth left. The *New England Journal of Medicine* reported [5] that the Merck Corporation instructed its salespeople to mislead physicians about the cardiovascular toxicity of its arthritis drug, Vioxx. Eli Lilly & Co. had its salespeople downplay the safety issues of Zyprexa, its star antipsychotic drug.[6] One might assume Lilly was adequately chastened when forced to pay out $1.2 billion dollars to thirty-one thousand damaged patients in Alaska. But no, that was only a cost of doing business: in 2007 Zyprexa earned Lilly $4.76 billion.

Business has so thoroughly permeated healthcare that more people make their living from diseases than die from them. Diabetes, for example, is a huge industry as well as a medical disorder.[7] For the last half-dozen years, many type 1 (insulin-dependent) diabetics have worn a tiny digital pump at their waist that delivers precise insulin doses under their skin. This gadget frees them from sticking their fingers and testing their blood sugar several times daily, calculating their dose, and finally injecting themselves. When these pumps first appeared, they were affordable. Now they cost seven thousand dollars and up, as manufacturers continually add bells and whistles: designer colors, bilingual talking pumps, minute-by-minute LED glucose level readouts. The pumps require accessories like hundred-dollar monitor probes that must be replaced weekly, disposable tubing, and ten daily test strips. Then there's the insulin—just a few dollars thirty years ago, but since most insulin is now patent-protected it can cost more than four thousand dollars annually.

The number of Americans diagnosed with diabetes has been increasing 50 percent every decade. Consequent expenditures could double by 2030, according to estimates by the U.S. Centers for Disease Control and Prevention. How many of us see this prophecy as an urgent invitation to develop prevention strategies and cheap, simple treatments, and how many see it as an opportunity to reap huge profits from sickness?

Screening for disease generates massive revenue, even when it's ineffectual. A recent study [8] involving 270,000 patients, published by the *Journal of the National Cancer Institute,* showed that while newer breast-imaging technologies (digital and computer-aided mammography, magnetic resonance imaging, and ultrasound) were believed to detect breast cancer at earlier stages, that hasn't turned out to be the case. They don't detect cancer earlier, but they do make mammography more expensive. Between 2002, when more advanced imaging became popular, and 2009, the cost went from $44 per patient to $63, and the cost of studies to follow up inconclusive results went from $32 to $43. Medicare's payment for these services rose from $666 million to $962 million, a 44 percent increase, while patients enjoyed no measurable benefit.

The chief medical officer of a huge healthcare organization pointed out that his hospital could make five thousand dollars from every free prostate cancer screening it offered, thanks to the ensuing biopsies, treatments, and follow-up care, some of which is unnecessary.

A study published in *Health Affairs* found that medical groups that sent specimens to their own labs ordered 72 percent more tests than groups that used independent facilities. That could be a legitimate practice, except that group-owned labs turned up fewer abnormalities than independent labs did.

Such practices begin to skirt the edge of criminality. A hospital chain based in Naples, Florida, allegedly kept scorecards [9] on its doctors. Those who admitted at least half of the elderly patients they saw in the emergency department were color-coded green. The names of doctors who admitted less than half were coded yellow, and failing physicians were red. Every day the scorecards were posted where all emergency room doctors could see them. Elsewhere in those establishments, docs were pressured to admit inappropriate patients, such as infants whose temperature was 98.7 degrees for a "fever." The U.S. Justice Department has joined eight separate whistle-blower lawsuits in six states against this chain.

No one's feasted at the trough more luxuriously than medical insurance corporations. This probably isn't news to you, so I'll offer only a single example: Aetna Insurance profited $31 billion in 2008. In 2010 it paid its CEO $24 million.

Even ostensibly humane advances are vulnerable to profiteering. For example, docs have long complained that perpetually mounting paperwork detracts from their time with and attention to patients. A recent study [10] concluded that two-thirds of a primary care physician's day was spent on clerical work that could be done by someone else. And patients, for their part, complain that doctors spend more time typing into their laptops than facing them.

A solution appeared recently in the form of the medical scribe. The scribe shadows the doctor, recording the patient's history and details of the exam, and writes progress notes, leaving the doctor free to simply practice medicine. These docs, who formerly spent late nights completing electronic patient records, now can relax with their families or get some sleep.

A win-win! The patient and doctor get to relate directly to each other, and the scribe gets paid for a useful service. Scribes typically earn eight to sixteen dollars hourly, and are usually paid by physicians. Yet they actually earn their own keep, since physicians say the time they save, three minutes per patient on average, *allows them to see up to four extra patients a day.* So I'm sorry, but that won't lengthen the seven-minute visit, only crowd the examining room a bit more.

Responding to public clamor for more personalized healthcare, some researchers are obliging, though in traditional biomedical style. They interpret "personal" not as the uniqueness of every soul, but as molecular specificity. They aim to identify individually unique molecular "biomarkers" found throughout patients' bodies in order to predict risk, make diagnoses, and select optimal treatments. So if you get tempted by a clinic's "personalized care" ad, ask what that phrase means.

Along with pushing products, the medical-industrial complex has convinced us that since healthcare is just another species of commerce, its difficulties and inequities can be remedied simply through accounting adjustments. As I followed the 2009 Congressional healthcare reform debate, I saw that testimony came exclusively from hospital administrators, insurance executives, and government officials, without a word from a single soul identified as a patient or practicing physician.

I was astonished at that omission, but younger folks I spoke with found that process sensible since during their lifetimes healthcare has always been a major industry. Lacking historical contrast, it also seems natural to them that after each patient visit it now costs doctors $58 to do the coding, billing, and collection just to get paid by insurance carriers. (Kids, that wasn't always so, either. My parents paid our pediatrician ten dollars cash for an office visit and fifteen for a house call, and that was that.)

Younger people might also see as a settled given that most doctors today are remunerated not by patients, but by private corporations or government agencies, usually according to "relative value units," RVUs. In primary care, an RVU is worth $35–45, depending on specialty and locale. If a fifteen-minute office visit is assigned an RVU of 0.8 and the doctor's paid $35 per RVU, that visit will earn the doctor $28. That's just for the visit. Value is added if the doctor performs a procedure. A thirty-minute colonoscopy, for example, is valued at around 6 RVUs, which would earn the doctor $210.

Suppose you'd been hospitalized for two days and received its bill while recuperating at home: twenty-eight thousand dollars. After you've regained consciousness, you conclude the total must be a decimal point off.

But it's not a mistake. The bill is correct if you accept its numbers. But press hospital administrators about the charges, and they'll admit they pulled them out of the air. (That practice apparently works well: tax-exempt "not-for-profit" hospitals are generally hugely profitable.) The March 4, 2013, edition of *TIME* magazine was devoted entirely to explaining why hospital bills are so ridiculously high [11]. The author, journalist Steven Brill, revealed that administrators assign a dollar amount to every service, from a heart transplant to dispensing an aspirin, and store those numbers in a software program called "Chargemaster." Every hospital maintains its list, and prices vary from institution to institution. Like car manufacturers' "recommended sticker prices," they're not numbers engraved in concrete, only the opening bid. Hospitals aren't eager to tell you that, but once you're aware of it, feel free to negotiate your hospital bill as you would a car price.

Start low. An outfit called Nerdwallet [12] compared the compensations hospitals accepted for knee surgery at a dozen San Francisco Bay Area hospitals. Medicare paid, on average, 27 percent of what these hospitals billed. Sure, Medicare takes advantage of the economics of scale, but nevertheless *took a 73 percent discount*. So don't be cowed by your thirteen-page Chargemaster bill. Multiply the grand total by 0.27 and make your offer. The hospital might not accept it, but at least it will begin a constructive discussion.

Dominated by business considerations, today's medical economics encourages doctors to *do*, to perform a colonoscopy or spinal tap or liver biopsy or stomach stapling. When they comply, they satisfy patients (who've learned to expect and even demand procedures), raise their own income, and as a bonus add momentum to the flywheel of commerce. For simply sitting and talking with patients, doctors are paid less or not at all. While they're loathe to do unindicated procedures, the financial incentive can push an undecided doc over the edge.

Medical students are at best dimly aware of the industrial mill they're entering. Imagine yourself in training, with altruistic stars in your eyes. Fifteen years later, when you're still struggling to pay off your six-figure education loan and your kids are applying for even larger loans of their own, your clinic manager informs you your last-quarter RVUs fell short. Now you'll need to see eight people hourly rather than six. Having fantasized yourself an independent professional, you realize you're actually an assembly-line chemical engineer, and it hurts. A 2007 survey by the physician-recruiting firm Merritt Hawkins indicated that half of a thousand doctors queried would not recommend their profession to their children. That's shocking enough, but a similar poll five years later by the Doctors Company, the nation's largest malpractice insurer, reported that 90 percent of five thousand physicians stated they were unwilling to recommend healthcare as a profession.

Most docs resent being manipulated by employers whose bottom line is the bottom line. They'd rather act from their clinical judgment and at a humane pace, but for many, overseen by managers attuned only to cash flow, that window has closed. I don't say this to paint commerce as unduly venal, for corporations are legally obliged to maximize investors' returns. *The question is whether healthcare should be a business at all* or, as it is in most of the developed world, a public service like education, policing, and firefighting.

CHAPTER 6

How to Be a Doctor

I was at a party with my friend Abe. When a woman asked him the extent of his education, he replied, "I have a master's in political science." Then she asked me. I said, "I'm an MD." Get it? Abe *has* a master's, I *am* an MD.

Medical students don't learn medicine like electricians learn wiring. We study our craft, to be sure, but learn also how to *be* a doctor. We absorb that role into our personhood, and in the style our culture prefers, the biomedical scientist. To understand the slow transformation of a young adult who wishes to heal people into an emotionally detached, dispassionate clinician, you'll need a brief tour of medical training.

On Day One, two parallel curricula crank up. The one that continues through residency is medicine. The longer—actually lifelong—course consists of steady induction into an exclusive subculture.

Doctors-in-training learn a worldview that values fact and logic far over subjective considerations like emotion. In fact, stature in the medical community rests largely on demonstrated devotion to objectivity. This focus is biomedicine's strength, and, as we'll see, its weakness.

We learn a special language. If you're not a doctor, eavesdrop on a medical discussion. For all you comprehend, you might as well be observing the Albanian parliament. We docs learn what to say, how to say it, and what not to say. We learn to see patients' pathologies, what's gone wrong, while relatively ignoring their normalities. And we tend to socialize with our professional peers, which continually reinforces our objectivist style. Our years of sequestered training result in a kind of cultural emigration. We eventually inhabit a world distinctly different from that of non-medical people.

If scientific subjects are biomedical training's lyrics, "How To Be A Doctor In This Particular Society" is its tune. Almost any American physician will agree that his or her education's background Muzak was characterized by several consistent and persuasive themes.

Rigid hierarchy

Freshman medical students are wretches akin to army recruits. Sophomores and juniors are noticed, but mainly as annoyances. Seniors, having attained a summit of sorts, are mere gofers for interns, who, in turn, are nameless drudges to resident physicians. At the pyramid's apex, the chair of the department glows with success while fretting about the associate professors clawing at his or her ankles.

Hierarchies invite internal abuse, which inevitably flows downhill. As a senior student, I saw a resident loudly upbraid my intern. An hour later, that same intern berated me for a minor omission. And that evening, I'm sorry to say, I joked with my roommates about how dirt-ignorant one of my patients was.

Feelings of inadequacy

There's far more for doctors-in-training to know than anyone can possibly learn. In addition, what was so yesterday may be obsolete today. In a probably apocryphal story, a medical school dean advised his new graduates, "I'm sorry, but a third of what we've taught you is incorrect. We just don't know which third."

Little wonder that students perennially feel deficient. Medical rounds in teaching hospitals are in part a compensatory ritual in which students and doctors recite scholarly references as claims of adequacy. Called "roundsmanship," the practice is defined as:

whoever's lacking here, it sure isn't me. Years of such defensiveness can breed a feigned confidence a tick short of arrogance.

Overwork and sleep deprivation

Ripping along on caffeine all night to prepare for next morning's freshman physiology exam is grueling, but only tepid practice for junior year, when the student will see patients around the clock. In addition, sleeplessness dulls the edge of intellect, leaving the student ready, even longing, to accept instruction unquestioningly.

American media revives the overwork issue as regularly as a cicada cycle. When we discover that a surgical resident about to operate on us hasn't slept since St. Swithin's Day, we jump off the table, write letters to editors, and call for Congressional hearings. Headlines blare outrage for a week. Then the issue burrows underground again for a decade. That this pattern has persisted so long and with so little reform suggests that we as a society believe healers *ought to* overwork. Of all the ways we could see healing, we choose to regard it as a zero-sum game, the patient's improvement roughly equivalent to the healer's depletion.

Overwork isn't confined to medical circles. It qualifies as a national trait. To paraphrase Calvin Coolidge, "The business of America is busyness." While every country in the European Union has at least four legally mandated weeks of paid vacation, the United States hasn't a single legally required paid holiday. The average U.S. employee clocks 20 percent more hours than counterparts in Germany or France.

We're obligate go-getters who speak of leisure as "kicking back," hardly a tranquil metaphor. Our medical training, having expertly prepared doctors to lead the pack of *Workaholicus americanus*, leaves us with hardly a handle on any notion of not-doing. My physiology professor, for example, taught that a muscle's sole function is contraction, that is, work. When a student objected that a muscle can't possibly contract without first relaxing, he said, "Relaxing? But that's not doing anything at all."

So do something, and do it now, "stat," and when you're finished, draw that blood down in room 121. Then find something else to do. Thinking, wondering, and chatting with patients might be virtuous, but it's extraneous to the task at hand. This hustle-bustle pays off later, in practice, as third parties pay for active procedures and not for simply listening to and comforting patients.

Unhesitating dedication

When medical students' personal needs compete with training obligations, they're reminded that a physician's devotion must be practically monastic (an apt term, as the non-medical are often referred to as "lay" people). By their third year, students accept that time with family, non-medical educational opportunities, and other deep interests must remain a remote vision.

One of my classmates, an Orthodox Jew, said he couldn't be available to work on Saturdays, the Sabbath. The dean had encountered that before. He reached into his files and showed the student a letter he'd secured from a rabbi stating that "saving lives" justified working on the Sabbath.

I'm not suggesting that medical students should come and go by whim, but if they're to comprehend patients, they need as much exposure to non-medical as medical life. The current style has them spending what sparse off-time they can glean either hermetically studying or restricting themselves to the tight circle of their classmates and its pervasive objectivist atmosphere.

Clinical distance

In my training, bedside rounds were exactly that, and not "patientside" rounds. Discussions were so abstract that the bed may as well have been empty. The patient was like a token in a game, a marker representing the actual situation. In many teaching hospitals, patients are referred to as "clinical material."

That may seem unconscionably impersonal, but students are led to such views in palatable increments from their first day, when, in an enduring tradition, the anatomy lab technician whips the sheet off a cadaver. In a way it's reasonable, as many students have never seen a dead body before, and over their career they'll see more than they'd like.

This first "patient" conveys another message, too, biomedicine's concept of patient as object. Of course, our first patient could have been a living, squirming one, but that variety is too complex to study through an objective lens. Live people, after all, need emotional appreciation, while cadavers make no subjective demands at all.

The cadaver ritual is closely accompanied by the "White Coat Ceremony" that almost all American medical schools now conduct. The initial donning of that professional emblem is meant to solemnize the physician role, especially its foundation in compassion. The ceremony's subtext is, "You're entering not just any job, but a calling that entails deep trust. You'll have access to people's bodies and souls. You'll be with them at birth and death and life's other mysteries. You'll encounter suffering that will test you daily. Go now, and grow."

That's a noble instruction, but schools don't generally address the "how" of it, so the coat ultimately signifies little more than role separation, an unhealthy dynamic that invites patients to idealize doctors and devalue their own knowledge. The irony would horrify the ceremony's creators. (In many hospitals, coat length indicates status—the longer the coat, the higher up the pyramid its wearer.)

While a student wears the white coat, the implicit biomedical message informing it may as well be, "A sick person is an intricate gadget on the fritz. Your task is to determine the problem and fix it. We'll show you how to do that. The patient's emotions or any wider perspective aren't your business. Don't think about whether this condition might actually be normal for this person, why he or she got sick, how a different lifestyle might have led elsewhere, how the person's race or income might have made a difference, or whether your practice enables pathogenic behavior rather than enhancing health. Just do your job: fix the gadget."

Opportunity is lost here, since in no other calling do we encounter the human condition so plainly. We docs witness plenty of suffering, and also kindness, joy, beauty, and justice. You know you're practicing well if you're in an almost continual state of amazement. Physician and poet William Carlos Williams observed, "To treat a man as something to which surgery, drugs, and hoodoo applied was an indifferent matter; to treat him as material for a work of art somehow made him come alive to me."

Biomedical chauvinism

Doctors learn that today's biomedicine was midwifed by Abraham Flexner and his patrons in the early twentieth century. And before that? Not much: bleeding, cupping, a few herbs, cathartics, and emetics. They're not educated about Hôtel Dieu's healing atmosphere or Dr. Trudeau's sanitarium because those were just styles, not scientific technologies.

The medical examination itself has begun to seem a relic of pre-digital yesteryear. When it's performed at all these days, it's partial and perfunctory. This despite the insistence of physician-author Abraham Verghese and other respected medical instructors that a thorough physical exam can diagnose accurately and more rapidly than thousands of dollars worth of high-tech tests. Further, Verghese writes, the exam can be a profound healing ritual.[1]

"Rituals are about transformation, the crossing of a threshold, and in the case of the bedside exam, the transformation is the cementing of the doctor-patient relationship, a way of saying: 'I will see you through this illness. I will be with you through thick and thin.' It is paramount that doctors not forget the importance of this ritual."

Medical students might welcome some of the old-fashioned skills Verghese recommends. They know docs didn't always have one wrist cuffed to a laptop and the other to an MRI machine. They've heard of more leisurely practices, such as house calls, sitting on the bed, staying for tea, and seeking the wider story. The style might actually enjoy a revival, if only instructors weren't too rushed themselves to model slowing down.

Some medical schools offer exposure to the non-biomedical disciplines called "alternative" or "complementary." Tens of millions of Americans, along with two-thirds of cancer patients, utilize acupuncture, massage, homeopathy, chiropractic, naturopathy, and other disciplines, finding them more generous with time, more cognizant of individuality, and often more personable. Yet medical educators still consider these practices the minor leagues, as they're not science-based, and only a rare doctor uses them in practice. When a patient informs a doctor, "I'm seeing an acupuncturist," a common lukewarm reply is, "Fine. I don't think it'll hurt." (Curiously, while much of the general public uses alternative treatments, the proportion is higher among doctors' family members.)

Youthful compliance

The conventional explanation for why there are so few older medical students is that their practice life will necessarily be shorter. A deeper reason is that having already half-filled their learning bucket, they're thought too old to learn much, which can also mean they've learned to think critically and will ask

embarrassing questions. In any case, students in their more mal-
leable early- and mid-twenties most readily memorize the syllabus.

Inadequate curriculum

Social change affecting healthcare has been colossal since today's
senior instructors graduated. A 2013 editorial in *San Francisco
Medicine Journal* [2] named a dozen topics indispensable in modern
practice yet neglected in training. Its co-authors, Dr. Philip Lee
and Dr. Gordon Fung, of the University of California San Francisco
School of Medicine, and SFMS Associate Executive Director Steve
Heilig, listed:

- Addiction
- Nutrition and complementary therapies
- Sexuality
- Pain
- End-of-life care
- Physical fitness
- Medical ethics
- Violence
- Environmental health
- Health policy
- The "business" of medicine
- Physicians' own well-being

As students inhabit this limited, limiting, and compelling
ambiance year after year, few don't eventually succumb to it. They
graduate into the wider world as experts in objective medical
science, but at the cost of knowing themselves and those they'll

serve. Their conversion from altruistic pre-meds into biomedical scientists, their slant toward fact and away from feeling, seeing pathology while ignoring normality, is so gradual—and so reasonable, really—that they hardly notice it.

The way we doctors come to see the world, then, isn't simply a preferred professional view. To us, it's the way things actually are. It's who I am and I'll resist persuasion otherwise.[3]

CHAPTER 7

Being a Doctor

Well-trained biomedical physicians halt infections, optimize cardiac outputs, properly set broken limbs, and much more. These are good things to do, and are essentially engineering skills. But genuine doctoring differs from engineering in that a patient isn't a cogwheel or an I-beam. Each is a world of meaning and emotion—hurting, disoriented, and vulnerable. Failure to attend to these invisible insides short-changes the patient and erodes the doctor as well. That which first attracted the doc to medicine will slowly leak away, and the head's vision will come to dominate the heart's.

Many years ago, I went with my wife, Ronnie, to hear former *Saturday Review* editor Norman Cousins speak at a university medical center. In his bestselling book, *Anatomy of an Illness*, he described his experience with a galloping case of ankylosing spondylitis, a painful savaging of the spine.

Cousins wrote that he was dissatisfied with his hospital stay, so moved to a four-star hotel next door at a fraction of the cost. He persuaded his doctors to visit him there and to restrict blood-drawing to a single daily stick. Discontinuing his medications, he treated himself instead with megadoses of vitamin C and laughter in the form of Marx Brothers and Candid Camera films. With this regimen, his spondylitis evaporated, a fact his doctors' testimonials corroborate.

Cousins told his story to this audience of physicians, nurses and students, and then called for questions. A doctor stood and asked, "Mr. Cousins, laughter is certainly a positive thing, but how could we devise a double-blind, controlled study in order to know objectively whether it aids healing?"

Giggling arose from the crowd. Obviously this Cousins fellow was no scientist. Ronnie's usually aristocratic manners couldn't abide the disrespect. She stood up beside me and called to the questioner, "If you don't know right now that laughter aids healing, there's something seriously wrong with you."

I agree with her. The doctor had dropped a chunk somewhere along the way, but a chunk of what? Common sense? A feeling for people? Whatever it is, it's a prominent loss. If he suspects Ronnie was right about him, he'd be wise to keep that to himself, since biomedicine doesn't take kindly to practitioners' vulnerabilities.

A physician friend was teaching communication skills to a roomful of his colleagues. In one exercise, he asked them to identify some personal ache or pain. A symptom of some sort was necessary for the exercise, yet no participants admitted to any.

"Well," he said, "can you remember one you had in the past? Can you imagine feeling it now as it was then?"

Most went along with this, but one doc said he was unable. "Okay," my exasperated friend said. "Is there anything in your life that gives you pain or grief or any kind of unhappiness?"

"Ah, well . . . maybe I could be earning more."

Another friend who facilitated a support group for physicians in Maryland told me members obsessed about confidentiality. She said they wouldn't have hidden an extramarital affair as carefully as they did their attendance at those meetings. They insisted repeatedly that not only wasn't a single word to leave the room—a standard practice anyway—but that no one outside the group was even to learn of their participation. They were afraid others would assume the group was an Impaired Physician Program which addresses suspected incompetence due to alcoholism, drug dependence, senility, or criminality.

If the appearance of vulnerability is unadvisable in biomedicine, death is flat-out unspeakable. Many years ago, a physician on our local medical staff developed a virulent illness and died within the month. Afterward, at our weekly lunch rounds, no one mentioned him. I thought maybe I'd missed a collegial memorial gathering, but no, that wasn't the case. Since then, other docs have died, too, without ever a public word from their fellows. Docs mourn like anyone does, but not at work. This is a strange prohibition, since birth and death are part of medicine's stock-in-trade.

Ironically, aversion to subjective processes like emotion and imagination inhibits medical progress. Several years ago I attended a dermatology lecture. Showing a photographic slide, the presenter said, "This illustrates the kind of lesion you get with Type A skin." With the next slide, she said, "This one, though, is more characteristic of Type B skin."

On and on, Type A and Type B. Finally, one physician asked, "Excuse me, but I've never heard of Type A and B skin. Where is this in the medical literature?"

The dermatologist looked shocked. "It's not in the literature. It's my fantasy."

The room exploded as physicians, livid that their time was wasted, shook their fists and stormed out. The presenter called after them, "What's the matter? Don't you fantasize?"

Of course they fantasize, but, like mourning, not within scientific practice.

That's bizarre, since science necessarily begins with fantasy. Is there actually a "Type A" and "Type B" skin? We have no idea, but it wouldn't occur to us to explore that or any notion until we wonder about it. Albert Einstein, the archetypical scientist, hardly ever entered a laboratory. His revelations gelled while he lay on his back in his sailboat on a Swiss lake, daydreaming. "The most beautiful experience we can have is the mysterious," he wrote.

"It is the fundamental emotion which stands at the cradle of true art and true science." Einstein's colleague, Nobel physicist Max Planck (1858–1947) extended that thought: "Science cannot solve the ultimate mystery of nature. And that is because, in the last analysis, we ourselves are a part of the mystery that we are trying to solve."

The biomedical preference for fact over subjectivity can be useful in, say, suturing a wound or calculating a dose, but can be hell on relationships with patients. When I was in standard practice, I prided myself on my ability to communicate. I explained everything to patients, with splendid clarity. In fact, I was "a legend in my own mind," as author Jay McInerney put it, until a few patients offered me feedback quite the opposite. "You talk a good game," said one, "but you're an awful listener." I realized that while I was busy picking through patients' narratives for diagnostic clues, I was deaf to their stories, and couldn't recognize an emotion if it bit me.

Unhealthy as that imbalance is for doctors' relationships with patients, it injures them as well. Try this experiment: during the next week, concentrate only on fact and logic while avoiding emotions, including your own. If you notice that this abridges your interactions a bit, imagine what a few decades of it will do.

Look up doctors' rates of burnout, divorce, drug dependence, alcoholism, and other sorrows. Male doctors have a 40 percent higher suicide rate than the general population, and female doctors a shocking *130 percent* higher. If the most prominent criticism of biomedicine is its enormous expense, the saddest is that it abuses its own practitioners by shriveling their softer human qualities.

If you're not a physician, imagine continually needing to appear objective and emotionally uninvolved with the suffering people you serve. The effort makes me recall a century-old photo of boys at the beach. Wearing the dark wool swimsuits of the time, each stiffly flexes his biceps along with his jaw. I want to ask them, "Are you tired of holding that pose?"

CHAPTER 8

Doctors and Suffering

Late one night, five ambulances screamed into our emergency department carrying many parts of three patients, the ghastly results of a bombing. Horror paralyzed me, but then I remembered: This is your job; stuff your feelings and get busy. And I did. Medical work sometimes requires parking emotions, acting cleanly from fact rather than feeling.

Another reason medical people require emotional distance is self-protection. At least that's what's said: If they didn't defend themselves from the suffering that permeates every hour of their career, they'd be chronically distraught. Their trained focus on fact shelters them from practice's daily emotional storm.

It's a porous refuge, though. Imagine a judge futilely advising the jury, "Ignore that outburst." If I make my living beside patients' crises, often with my fingers inside their bodies, it's preposterous for me to claim I'm not emotionally involved with them. Let's face it: We who wade through suffering absorb it like butter into hot toast. Once it's in us, what do we do with it?

Doctors (along with others who professionally encounter suffering, including firefighters, police, and military personnel) must choose between either feeling the pain inherent in their work or somehow avoiding it. Toward the latter goal we've devised a variety of strategies.

Last year I was chatting with a pathologist who told me one of his specialty's advantages was patient contact.

"That's unusual," I said. "Pathologists are notorious medical homebodies. How exactly do you contact patients?"

He said, "Well, sometimes I'll read a tissue slide and it doesn't quite add up. But when I go to the ward and read the patient's chart, things almost always make sense."

I was puzzled. "And you see the patients, then?"

Now he looked puzzled. "See the patients? Why would I do that? All I need is the chart."

I was with another physician, a gentle rheumatologist whose patient was crying in pain. If the thought balloon over his head were legible, it would have read, "My God, this poor young woman is suffering horribly. I want to get up and just hold her. On the other hand, that wouldn't be professional."

He wrung his hands, his two sides struggling with one another. In the end, he stayed put, resumed an impassive face, and wrote her a prescription for a more potent painkiller. Afterward, I asked him how he'd felt.

"Ripped in half."

"Ripped in half? How do you mean?"

"I don't want to talk about it," he answered. "I need to get back to work."

Some physicians choose to regard feelings as irrelevant static. An oncologist at a cancer center where I facilitated support groups questioned the legitimacy of my work.

"There's no way to measure its efficacy," he said. "Give a hundred patients with infections the right antibiotic, and eighty-five will be cured. That's solid numbers. But can you apply anything like that to a support group?"

"Well, there's more to life than what can be measured."

"Like?"

Okay, he asked for it. Glancing at a photo on his desk, I said, "How do you know you love your wife?"

Uh oh. I think I might've touched a nerve. He sputtered, frothed, and walked out. He continued his work, and I mine.

What should we docs do with the agony we can't help but soak up? I saw a video that shed light on this question. Filmed in several major cancer centers, it depicted oncologists role-playing patients in a mock support group. The only coaching they'd been given was the assignment of a diagnosis. Their play was in three acts. In the first act, these "patients" ad-libbed about what it was like to have cancer. After a short intermission, they returned to their places, but now in makeup. Bald, pale, and bruised, pushing IV poles, they expressed tribulations of treatment. After another intermission they returned again, surprised to find one seat empty. In this third act, they talked about death and dying.

Considering the complaints I hear from patients about cold, impersonal, uncaring doctors, this video startled me: the oncologists portrayed patients with astounding nuance. When we doctors seem dispassionate, then, it's not because we don't notice suffering. On the contrary, we do indeed feel your pain, in fine detail. Since we don't know how to dissipate it, it inhabits us, tenaciously.

We suffer what neurologists would call "expressive aphasia": we comprehend but are unable to speak, in this case to express emotion. We have feelings galore. We fall in love, laugh at jokes, and weep at memorials, but expressing emotions within our professional setting would give us away as mere pretenders to the institution of objective biomedicine.

We repress not only feelings absorbed from suffering patients, but our own emotions as well, and that begs trouble. Researchers in the Mayo Clinic recently found that 45 percent of more than seven thousand doctors surveyed reported experiencing at least one symptom of burnout, almost double the rate of other working adults. The report blamed several factors, including a decline in the sense of meaning that physicians derive from their work, and difficulty integrating personal and professional life. "Unfortunately," the report concluded, "little evidence exists about how to address this problem."

Oh, come now. We address burnout like we would any difficulty, first by noticing what we feel. Frustrated? Angry? Sad? Once consciously recognized, the emotion will drive our response. ("Emotion," "motivation," and "motion" share the same root.) If instead of recognizing how we feel, we let it churn amorphously inside us, we won't act, only grumble about patients, colleagues, hospitals, Medicare, and other handy targets. Then, gritting our teeth, we'll return to work. That advice, "Physician, heal thyself," pops up again: if we wish to treat our patients' suffering, we can do so only to the extent we address our own.

CHAPTER 9

When Doctor Meets Patient

I n the late 1970s I offered a community college course called "Philosophy of Health." That title sounds dry now, even to me, and of course, no one came. When I added "Holistic" to the title, this being California, we couldn't find enough chairs. We spent one session role-playing. People paired off, and for five minutes one partner took the part of "patient" and the other, "doctor." Then they switched roles. Finally, we talked about it.

Each time we did this exercise, students commented on the polar differences they'd discovered. The composite review was, "When I played doctor, I felt intelligent and competent. I felt in control, or at least that I needed to look that way. I also felt inordinately responsible, pushed to do something, anything. I was surprised that it wasn't pleasant. But neither was the patient role, where I felt relatively ignorant, dependent, even physically small."

The role disparities conspire a vertical patient–doctor connection, like that of student and teacher. That fits popular culture's glorification of physicians as brilliant action heroes saving patients. Consider television's Dr. Konrad Steiner ("Medic: the eye of an eagle, the heart of a lion, the hand . . . of a woman."[1] In fact, for an eye-opening tour of medicine of that time, the 1950s, watch the whole program), Dr. Ben Casey, Star Trek's Dr. "Bones" McCoy, and Dr. Gregory House. We never see any of these champions quietly sitting with a patient, listening, or contemplating because they're can-do, caffeinated live wires.

Suddenly realizing that the correct diagnosis is tetanus, they run to the bedside, push the intravenous antitoxin, and the patient soon returns happily home.

Pop culture convinces us that high-tech docs not only cure all tetanus, but can turn away the Grim Reaper indefinitely. This flattering Hollywood fiction has us make tragically unreal demands on doctors. For example, a study of how cardiopulmonary resuscitation—CPR—is portrayed on television found that it was successful in three-quarters of the cases. A study of ninety-nine thousand actual CPR cases found, though, that only two hundred twenty-eight patients, *a fifth of 1 percent*, were pulled from death into a relatively normal life. The rarity of success doesn't mean we shouldn't try, only that surreal expectations beget disappointment.

The wishful thinking flame is fanned by infomercials touting the latest "breakthroughs," and magazine ads advising us to ask our doctor if a daily dose of Panacea™ will repair our lives. Inundated with messages suggesting that doctors can cure whatever ails us, anything patients might contribute seems negligible in comparison. In any case, the massive quantity of these ads feeds the myth that technology is a miraculous fix-all.

Though patients romanticize biomedicine's capabilities, they sorely miss plain old comforting. My friend Richard broke his hand and suffered facial injuries in an auto accident. He was promptly triaged in a trauma center, his lacerations were stitched, and then he was left alone. Lying on a gurney, he discovered his condition was rosy compared to others brought in lacking limbs or heartbeat, so he resolved to wait patiently. Fourteen hours later, a nurse put an ice pack on his hand.

While convalescing, Richard told me, "A trauma center can be too hectic a place for personal attention. I understand that. Yet even Walmart employs greeters. I had injuries that needed attention, but more than anything else, *I* was hurting, too: me, my insides, the part that doesn't show. I was frightened, disoriented, and vulnerable. Even a volunteer hanging out with me for a few minutes would have made a world of difference."

That simple and sensible suggestion doesn't require any healthcare revolution, only the slightest fine-tuning. Polly, a nurse's aide in our emergency department, was our in-house comforter. Well into her sixties, she'd cheerfully forgotten most of the medicine she'd learned, but she had The Touch. When an ambulance delivered a young motorcyclist who'd suffered fractures and was quaking with pain and fear, we made room for Polly to squeeze in at the gurney. She took his bloody hand in hers, smiled warmly at him, and said, "Honey, you're a mess. But we're going to get you fixed up." He actually smiled.

Patients and doctors maintain languages, outlooks, emotional tones, and goals so dissimilar that when they convene, they may as well be Inuit meeting Tuareg. Their communication will snag, and they'll behave in ways incomprehensible to each other.

- A doctor felt it was time to talk with her patient about hospice care, but she delayed because, she said, "I didn't want to scare her." The patient said, "I wanted to ask the doctor about hospice care, but I didn't want her to think she'd failed, so I didn't bring it up."

- A doctor summoned a patient into his office to discuss test results. "After he said the C word," the patient said, "I didn't hear a thing. I'm sure my eyes glazed over. But he kept talking and talking . . ." The doctor said, "I sometimes wonder why I spend so much time trying to educate patients. Half the time they're not listening."

- A man told his doctor he was in pain. The doctor recommended an over-the-counter pill. After that drug proved ineffective, the doctor explained, "He just told me he hurt. If he'd told me his pain level was nine out of ten, I would've prescribed something stronger."

- A woman asked her doctor how serious her condition was. The doctor told her to just let him worry about it. At home, she said, "Well, fine. Maybe he can turn it off, but I can't. In fact, worry is all I'm really sick with now."

- A man said, "If only the doctor had admitted he'd made a mistake, I'd have forgiven him. It's his stonewalling that made me sue him." The doctor said, "I felt terrible about what happened, but my lawyer told me not to talk about it."

- A patient complained that her doctor's nurse informed her of her cancer diagnosis with a message left on her answering machine on a Friday afternoon. "How can you leave a message like that? I couldn't even ask any questions about it until Monday morning." The doctor explained, "I think patients ought to get information right away."

- A woman freshly diagnosed with leukemia became extremely anxious. She called her doctor's office six to eight times daily with questions. The nurse courteously answered her first several calls, but soon felt burdened by the interruptions, and instructed the receptionist to say she was busy. The patient said, "They probably think of me as a difficult patient now." She was right. Yet no one in the office talked with her about her actual suffering, her anxiety.

- A patient's son asked the doctor to do everything possible for his dying dad. The doctor complied. "I thought if I told them that heroic measures would be futile," the doctor said, "I'd destroy their hope." After the man died, the son said, "I wish the doctor had told us treatment would only prolong Dad's suffering."

- "I'm concerned about my patients' emotions," said a doctor, "so I ask them if they feel stressed. If they say yes, I send them to a psychiatrist. If they say no, I leave them be. I've begun to wonder, though, if they even know if they're stressed."

- A patient told her doctor she wanted to try acupuncture and herbs before she'd accept standard oncology. The doctor said that wasn't a great idea since her life was on the line: "Most of the people I've seen go alternative are dead." The patient replied, "Look, it's my life, and I need to be in the driver's seat. How many of your chemo patients are also dead?"

Biomedicine's high-tech focus makes a poor orphan of its lowest-tech aspect, communication. Healthcare screams for the more extensive conversations that generate mutual clarity. Communication is a dicey proposition in even the easiest of situations. We sense some notion we'd like to express, select words that more or less describe it, then pass those words through the air to someone who tries literally to "make sense" of them. I marvel that a listener ever fully comprehends a speaker's message, but the challenge in healthcare is greater, since the patient is compromised, the doctor isn't much motivated to speak plain language, and the rush of practice pressurizes the transaction.

The difference between patient and doctor is starkly illuminated when both occupy a single body. In his book *When Doctors Become Patients,* Dr. Robert Klitzman, a Columbia University psychiatrist, relates his own experience along with those of more than seventy men and women who have known both ends of the stethoscope.

Klitzman's sister, Karen, worked in the World Trade Center, and died in the 9/11 attack. After the funeral, he couldn't get out of bed, and developed what felt like the flu. Though he's a psychiatrist, he resisted the view that he was depressed. Later, after acknowledging his illness, he found new insight into his patients. "I felt weak and ashamed," he writes, "and began to appreciate the embarrassment and stigma my patients felt."

Another doctor-patient Klitzman describes, a gastroenterologist who'd suffered abdominal pain, said, "I had no idea that when patients said *pain*, this is what they were talking about. It was so much beyond words."

Docs who become patients are uniformly surprised to find they're suddenly vulnerable and disoriented. This is an especially troubling predicament, since it's the opposite of their usual sensibility, and may account for their reputation as terrible patients. I don't wish sickness on my colleagues, but eventually most, like all people, will get sick, so when it happens I wish them insight.

Their practices might benefit from their illness experience, since it plunks them into the archetype of the "wounded healer," the doctor who can genuinely empathize because he or she has been there. Over the past thirty years, a half-dozen docs have joined cancer support groups I facilitated. Finding themselves in this disorienting role, each of them took me aside at some point and told me privately how stunned they were that the patient experience was so profound, and so different than what they'd believed. Two enjoyed enough remission to re-open their practices . . . and what different practices they were! These docs now couldn't bear to see more than six or eight patients daily. "In visits any shorter," said one, "how could I begin to know what they really need?"

A disease you haven't had, after all, is just another file in your frontal lobes, while one you've actually endured engraves itself on your soul. When I was a young physician who hadn't anguished much about anything, the suffering of my patients meant little to me. I hadn't a matrix of experience upon which to hang it.

A bumper-sticker comment that occasionally arises in our support group meetings is, "No one should be allowed to treat a disease they haven't had." Having had cancer may indeed be an asset in treating others' cancers, but to treat a person, the only requirement is to be one yourself.

One problem for docs is that putting themselves in patients' shoes challenges biomedical science's objectivity. For example, my friend Audrey told me, "I just spent two weeks with my mother. She's ninety and pretty disabled, but insists on living alone. So I regularly drive three hours to care for her and clean her place. I bring her to her doctor a couple of times a week. I love her and I'm happy to do it, but it takes its toll on me.

"As I drove home a few days ago, my back began hurting. By the next morning, it was pretty severe, so I arranged to see my doctor to get a prescription for something stronger than ibuprofen. When I saw him, I explained what my past two weeks had been like. I told him I thought my pain was from stress. He examined me and sent me for a CT scan.

"When I handed the order to the woman at the radiology desk, she said, 'You know, this will cost you a thousand dollars.' That was a shock. No way could I vote for a thousand dollars. I tore up the order, phoned the doctor's office, and told them no, I wasn't going to get the scan. I said my back hurt because I'd been carrying a huge burden, so I just wanted a strong painkiller and I'd wait the thing out. My doctor phoned a prescription to the pharmacy, and my pain's gone now.

"Why do they act that way? Why can't doctors just accept that sometimes patients actually know what they're talking about?"

Audrey's friends claim her doctor ordered the CT scan not for her welfare, but to avoid liability on his part by touching every conceivable base. Called "defensive medicine," this practice is thought to result in 20 to 30 percent of our national healthcare expense. Indeed, defensiveness is especially common when relationships between patients and their doctors are tenuous.

But as alarming to doctors as the fear of litigation is, equally potent is their fear of disappointing their profession by showing insufficient regard for scientific rigor.

After I related Audrey's story to a doctor friend, he surprised me by regarded me weirdly, as though thinking, "Hm. And here I'd thought all along this guy was competent."

"Wait a minute," he said. "Let's be responsible here. Sure, she was stressed, but what if she was hurting because of something in addition? How old is she? Has she been tested for osteoporosis? How do we know she doesn't have a pathologic fracture from a cancer metastasis?" He went on, impressively erudite.

One useful medical axiom advises, "When you hear hoofbeats outside, think of a horse before a zebra." That is, common events, like symptoms from stress, occur more often than uncommon ones like pathologic fractures. Yet if one mentions hoofbeats at a medical luncheon, every doc at the table will declare, "Right, but occasionally a zebra does show up." Not being Audrey's doctor, my friend has no need to practice defensively in her case. No, he offered his zebra list as roundsmanship, ritual dedication to science.

But wait, you say. What if he's right? Should Audrey worry that her pain is from something more serious than stress? Will she break a bone while working out? Are we ignoring an occult cancer?

Maybe. These are reasonable possibilities, however remote. But the issue here isn't diagnosis; it's confidence. Audrey was fairly sure—say 90 percent sure—that her back hurt simply from stress. Her doctor, though, felt uncomfortable settling for less than the 90 percent certainty biomedicine prefers and that a normal CT scan could have provided. Had he not recommended the scan, his colleagues would have sneered at his laxity, as though he'd ignored a spurting artery. Even though 100 percent certainty is impossible in this universe, biomedical scientists insist on getting as close as possible. And of course, enthusiastic vendors are standing by offering the assistance of their remarkable products. I predict that the thousand-dollar CT scan will soon be replaced by the *99.9-percent-accurate* megaholotropic scan—fictional at the moment, but a sure thing down the road—at five thousand dollars per. Since there's no end to high-tech development, we're permanently obliged to balance cost with confidence. Audrey satisfied herself with reasonable certainty at reasonable cost. Her decision included 10 percent faith, a function her doctor feels he must avoid.

Patients' and doctors' different ways of thinking pervade every aspect of practice. In a recent study, for example, researchers asked physicians which of two treatment scenarios they'd recommend for seriously ill patients. Scenario One carried a better chance of survival, but with dubious quality of life; call this choice "survival." Scenario Two, the "quality" choice, bore a lower chance of survival but better quality for the life remaining. The docs were more likely to opt for "survival" over "quality." Then they were asked which option they'd choose for *themselves*. They overwhelmingly went for "quality." Evidently we docs prefer objectively measurable outcomes such as survival time for our patients, but when we're the patient we heed our emotions.

The issue isn't whether we should treat our patients as they wish or as we wish, or as we'd treat ourselves. It's that the wisest choice will arise from patient and doctor together exploring the full range of options, and that demands the emotional honesty and trust of an intimate relationship.

CHAPTER 10

We Can Do Better

A question I regularly ask colleagues is, "Have you ever made an important medical decision that overrode your scientific data?"

If I ask it in a group, not a hand is raised. That hush is the medical equivalent of the Mafia's *omertà*, silence to protect the family. If it's just the two of us, though, they uniformly say yes and go on to relate an inspirational story, a tale of magic and miracle. Rarely do they regret their decision. They've learned that intuition isn't a hazy hunch, but a species of knowledge. Though we physicians are trained to downplay feelings, we utilize them anyway, albeit secretly and often unconsciously. Were we to use feelings diligently enough to become skilled with them, we'd find that they are the raw materials for healthcare's art.

The most universal emotional healing tool is the placebo. Healers around the world—shamans, mediums, witch doctors, *curanderos*—enact indigenous rituals to treat their patients' suffering by engaging their emotions and imaginations. Depending on where I'm sick, a healer will dance in the dust for me, wave a talisman, chant, pray, or prescribe me pills. Taking the ministration seriously, I then wonder if it's helped. So I feel around: does it hurt less now? How about *now*? Well, maybe it's helped a little, maybe more than a little.

Since it's the *wondering* that does the trick, placebos needn't be pills. In fact, we doctors are placebos. Our concerned, capable manner, starched white coat, and stethoscope amulet encourage patients to feel they're in good hands even before we physically treat them. And once applied, our treatment bears additional placebo potential. It's said that up to 40 percent of any drug's action results from placebo effect. Thus the "sugar pill"—with its appreciable efficacy and no attributable side effects—is very literally a wonder drug.

In the medical office, the receptionist, as initial contact and thus tone-setter, is a potential placebo. In fact, so is every element of the medical setting. There's a growing interest among hospital designers in promoting patients' sense of well-being by adding windows, brighter colors, welcoming furniture, evocative art, tastier food, and quieter rooms to the traditional somber, busy, green-walled institution.

Enhancing the atmosphere, by the way, isn't just an esthetic exercise, as hospitalization itself can discomfort patients so thoroughly that they're sometimes discharged in compromised shape and soon need readmission. In fact, patients older than sixty-five suffer such a high rate of troublesome, costly hospital readmission that Medicare has implemented incentives to reduce its occurrence.

A recent article in the *Journal of the American Medical Association* [2] defines "post-hospital syndrome" as increased illness susceptibility initiated by the stresses of hospitalization. The continual noise, lack of privacy, unexpected awakenings, examinations by strangers, and other common practices add up to a parade of assaults on one's person. The authors, Dr. Allan Detsky and Dr. Harlan Krumholz, ask the question we should have been asking the past century, "What would it take for hospitals to become truly healing environments?" These authors recommend adequate rest and nourishment, the elimination of unnecessary tests and procedures, and reduction of stress, surprises, and disruptions. Maybe the nuns who operated the Hôtel Dieu a thousand years ago knew something we're beginning to relearn.

The setting and tone of the medical transaction powerfully affect patients. Educators who realize this have taken practical steps to offer students useful tips: sit at the patient's level, make eye contact, acknowledge the patient's comments, touch when appropriate. Such suggestions, though valid, are actually simulations of compassion where the real thing would be more effective. Still, the strategy means well, and I've seen it gradually naturalize in some young docs.

The most tangibly therapeutic relationship is one that's genuinely intimate. In his book about navigating his own cancer, *Intoxicated by My Illness*, Anatole Broyard, the late *New York Times* literary critic, wrote, "I can imagine my doctor entering my condition, looking around at it from the inside like a benevolent landlord with a tenant, trying to see how he could make the premises more livable for me. He would see the genius of my illness. He would mingle his *dæmon* with mine; we would wrestle with my fate together . . ."

Obviously, this isn't a picture of a "provider" tendering "healthcare" to a "consumer." It depicts committed concern and emotional involvement. The closest comparison I can make is friendship. So when I hear, as I often do these days, "Can compassion be taught?" I think the more apt question is, "Can we un-teach emotional detachment?"

My friend Norm is a physician who decided that closer listening would reveal a patient's story beyond the symptoms. One afternoon he saw Milly, who had recently transferred to him from another doctor. She suffered from an autoimmune disease with arthritis that migrated around her body.

"Other doctors have had me on painkillers and steroids," Milly said. "How would you approach it?"

"Well, are you satisfied with those meds?"

"Yes and no. They're okay at treating my symptoms, but I'm pretty young and would rather not put up with their side effects the rest of my life. Do you think this is curable?"

"I don't know. Can you tell me more about what it's like to live with this?"

"It began about a year after I got married. My left hand started hurting, and the finger joints swelled up. I couldn't even get my ring off."

"A year after you got married . . . your ring . . ."

"So?"

"Well, that's just an unusual way to put it. Do you always mention your marriage and the onset of your illness in the same sentence?"

Milly paused. "Well, the truth is I've wondered about a connection, but that's not possible, is it?"

"I don't know. Tell me about your marriage."

In the privacy of the exam room, Milly told Norm the ways in which her union was unhappy. Whether that was actually connected to her illness or not, Norm realized, Milly viewed it as a significant issue.

He asked, "Have you spoken with anyone else about this?"

She looked at the floor. "No. Not even my husband. I can't tell him something like that. He'd think he caused my illness. That would destroy him."

"Milly," Norm said, "the fact that you imagine some link between your illness and your marriage seems important to me. No one can possibly know what actually caused your illness, but in any case you've told me you're not happy. Do you think that's worth exploring, say with a counselor?"

Milly did. Norm prescribed analgesic pills and small doses of a steroid to control her symptoms. She began to see a counselor weekly. After several visits, her husband joined her in therapy. They jointly concluded they probably never should have married in the first place. A few months after they separated, Milly's illness vanished..

The questions Norm asked Milly (Do you connect your illness with your marriage? How is your marriage, anyway?) are outside traditional medical boundaries. Early in my career, I would have considered them impertinent, even offensive, and would have asked just enough to attain my goal, a physical diagnosis. Norm, listening more than he spoke, tried to comprehend Milly's full situation, not just its medical aspect. Since treatment depends on diagnosis, what was Milly's diagnosis, after all, an autoimmune disease alone, or a physical disorder that proclaimed a troubled life?

Another example is Patricia, a family physician. Her patient, fifty-five-year-old Harry, was forty pounds overweight and suffered from type two diabetes. During the previous two years Patricia had had him on a medication that controlled his blood sugar. But she was getting frustrated.

"Sure, those pills work for Harry," she said, "but he wouldn't need them at all if he lost enough weight, and he knows that because I've told him till I was blue in the face. I wonder whether I'm helping some of my patients get healthier or, God forbid, helping them stay unhealthy."

A year earlier, she wouldn't have mentioned her feelings to any patient, but now she realized her frustrations with some of them were a daily pebble in her shoe. During Harry's next visit, Patricia said, "Look, Harry, you're doing okay, but I don't think it's a good idea either to keep you on drugs forever or to let you carry around this extra weight."

Harry pondered this. "You know I've tried and tried. I just can't keep the weight off."

"No one says it's easy, Harry, but it's getting down to no other choice. There are some reputable programs and counselors around. I know you've tried some, and I applaud you for that. But look, this is a matter of life and death. I have to tell you that."

"You think I'll die from this?"

"I don't know. But if you thought that was likely, would you behave differently?" She paused a moment, then found herself saying, "This is frustrating for me. I heard of a doctor who refuses to see smokers, and I can understand how she feels. She says treating them is only enabling their sick-making behavior."

"Are you going to fire me?"

"Of course not. I'm just trying to give you an idea of how important this is, not just to you, but to me, too. Harry, I'm tearing my hair out."

Harry left with his refill prescription, along with fresh sobriety about his situation. He read extensively on nutrition, joined a support group, dropped pounds slowly over the following months, and in a year no longer needed his diabetes meds. And Patricia, having expressed herself similarly to other patients, no longer tears her hair out. That is, she healed her own suffering by taking her emotions seriously.

Examples abound. My friend Frank, a family physician, assiduously stuffed his emotions connected with his practice. He expressed his dissatisfactions—burdensome paperwork, grueling hours, lost family time, underpayment, overregulation, and under-appreciation—to colleagues, but with a straight face, as though reciting a shopping list . . . until he finally fired a patient.

"I should have cut him loose decades ago," he said. "Whenever I saw his name on the appointment list I got a migraine. I don't know if he's a psychopath or passive-aggressive or an outright criminal, but he angers everyone around him.

"I'm amazed at myself for putting up with him so long. What was I thinking? I tried to be professional. Detached, unemotional. I don't know, maybe my self-image changed. One day when I was with him I thought, 'Excuse me, but evidently you think you're dealing with someone who gratefully accepts your crap.' I didn't actually say that, though. I just told him I wouldn't be his doctor anymore, and handed him the legal form. When he left, I felt like a boulder had been lifted off me.

"I think I understand better now why some women stay with abusive men. They say he didn't really mean it, they must've done something to provoke him, he was just having a bad day. Whatever rationalizations I'd made about this patient just evaporated one morning when a little voice inside me said, loud and clear, 'Guess what: you're being abused.'"

Norm, Patricia, and Frank don't practice on some other planet. The flavor of these patient contacts departed only slightly from that of standard medical visits. The difference is that these docs honored feelings—patients' and their own—as thoroughly as they value blood tests. Norm heard Milly's unhappiness, Patricia appreciated her own exasperation, and Frank acted effectively from appropriate anger.

A common criticism of addressing emotions along with facts is that it requires a longer appointment: I can't listen to your woes and weep along with you while a dozen other patients are waiting. Actually, though, it takes less time. An effective intervention can be a word or touch so fleeting that the practitioner doesn't even remember doing it. Besides, compare the total time of six impersonal, ineffective ten-minute visits with a single intimate visit of forty minutes.

The time issue is a red herring, anyway, since time is always a function of personal priorities. We docs will go more deeply with patients when we feel it's important enough, to them and to us. Anyone who wishes to be an instrument of healing must consider occasionally softening boundaries. Hopefully we can start to think of many more people as "Doctors Without Borders."

CHAPTER 11

Caregiver: The Invisible Patient

Ellen is in remission two months after treatment for lung cancer. Her only remaining symptom is anger at her husband, Eric, who's on the Internet most of his waking hours, seeking clinical trials and alternative treatments.

Recently she screamed at him, "You're gone, off in cyberspace! I hardly ever see you. Me, your wife, I'm here. Be with me!"

He answered, "I'd love to, but you won't be here long if you get a recurrence and we haven't found a cure."

Ellen has reminded Eric more than once that expert practitioners treat and monitor her, that he's unlikely to discover a resource they don't already know about, and that she misses him. Eric even admits that he's frantic in his attempts to save Ellen. He doesn't understand that his frenzy isn't about cancer or even Ellen, but his own treatable anxiety.

That is, Eric's a patient, too. He suffers his version of Ellen's cancer. As long as he continues to believe that Ellen is the sole patient, their torment will not resolve.

A common observation within cancer support groups is that caregivers can suffer more than the identified patient does. Yet in medical education circles, courses concerning caregivers are so rare that practitioners are not only unequipped to treat them, but lack any notion of caregivers' miseries. No wonder I've heard caregivers call themselves "invisible patients."

Those who care for sick people can experience the same intense anger, depression, confusion, and isolation that patients encounter. Left untreated, these emotions can bloom into physical disorders. Studies have found that caregivers are at risk for high blood pressure, impaired immunity, and cardio-vascular disease. Spousal caregivers age sixty-six or older have a 63 percent higher mortality rate than non-caregivers the same age.

When someone's sick, their house may as well be on fire, with every resident breathing the smoke. Partners are complexly affected, as they can be reluctant to reveal their pain, worry, and fatigue to their already-burdened mate. Children, who conjure every kind of magical thought, can believe their parent is sick because they neglected to put away their toys. Young adult children, just starting to build their lives, would rather not think about, let alone talk about, mortality. While some friends drop by with lasagna, others, worried or fearful, drop away.

My friend Fred, who cared for his wife Linda after she had elective surgery, told me, "I expected the work, but I sure didn't expect medical people to treat me like I wasn't there." Fred prepared meals for Linda, and re-prepared them when their ingredients repelled her. He bandaged her, emptied her bedpan, gave her sponge baths, and took calls.

Linda expressed her gratitude to Fred continually. Sometimes she couldn't say what she wanted, though, so Fred had to guess. A couple of times Linda's condition went south without her knowledge, so Fred had to keep constant watch. The requisite vigilance didn't leave much attention for his interests, sleep, or even rest.

Linda didn't do well on her post-op pain meds. Too small a dose left her in agony, while an adequate dose made her a vomiting wreck. A doctor friend suggested a different regimen, which made sense to Fred, so he called Linda's doctor's office.

The nurse said, "Sure, we can try that. You'll have to come by and pick up the prescription in person."

He hadn't slept much the previous night, so after Fred had driven thirty miles to the medical office, he looked like he'd been through a chipper. The receptionist asked, "How are you?"

"Pretty frazzled."

With that, the portcullis slammed down. No more eye contact with the receptionist. The nurse heard him, too, and suddenly remembered something she needed to do in another room. The doctor glanced up, then away, and disappeared. Fred got the prescription, though, and in the following days it proved effective.

On the drive home, Fred asked himself, "Why would they act like that? Did I frighten them? Don't they take some oath to relieve suffering?"

Bluntly, Fred wasn't their patient. Linda was. Previous contact revealed the staff to be caring people, but their behavior with Fred said, "Sorry you're frazzled, but you're not our responsibility."

Family members aren't the only caregivers whose suffering is regularly ignored. Consider professional caregivers, physicians.

Alan, a twenty-two-year-old man, told me of the time he learned his diagnosis of Hodgkins' lymphoma. "My parents came with me to that appointment. We all dreaded it," he said. "I was a senior in high school then. After I heard the word 'cancer,' my hearing turned off. The rest of the day I was a zombie. My mother didn't say a word, just began crying. And my father got angry. He stood up and his face got red and he yelled, 'No! No! This isn't supposed to happen!'

"What surprised me was the doctor. We were blown away. Gone. It should've been obvious to anyone that we weren't the doctor's audience anymore, but he went right on talking. He picked up a chart from his desk and pointed out lines on it, red ones creeping up and blue ones going down. He was so tense, so uptight that I guessed he needed to keep talking so he wouldn't just break down.

It couldn't have been easy for him. I mean, how would you like to give that kind of news to families every day? I once wanted to be a doctor, but now I know I could never handle stuff like that."

Among our stranger cultural views is that caregivers must appear composed for the patient's sake, and demonstrate selfless dedication. They're expected to devote unlimited hours to feeding, cleaning, comforting, accompanying, transporting, and advocating for their loved ones while disregarding their own lives, and to serve themselves a generous slice of guilt if they fall short of that ideal. It's as if they're to transfuse their own blood into the patient until they themselves are anemic.

It doesn't have to be that way. Caregiving can actually be synergistic: done well, both parties will feel better. That requires that caregivers get adequate nutrition, sleep, support, and time off.

They need appreciation, too, which needs to be distinguished from tribute. Appreciation simply honors what you do: "You take great care of Mom, and I can see how it tires you." Tribute, though, is hyperbole intended to fix your suffering and the speaker's guilt for not helping more: "You're Superwoman. You're another Mother Teresa. I could never do what you're doing." Like a sugar hit, it's delicious but wears off quickly.

We're only human. Compassion is ultimately draining, so must be spent judiciously. I recently experienced my first instance of compassion fatigue.[1] Several of my friends got seriously ill at the same time, and others died of illness and accidents. The air in our home began to reek of pain, and I couldn't smell it since I'm, well, a male, ever strong and capable. My wife pointed out that I was exhausted and was angering without provocation. I finally realized that I couldn't take on any more. I turned off the phone and ignored my email, and in a couple of days I smelled sweet again.

As caregivers, we shouldn't have to get sick in order to back off and take care of ourselves. We have the right and actually the obligation to do so. We need to check in often with a professional counselor, a support group, or a skilled friend, defined as someone who both listens well and feels comfortable telling us what we don't want to hear.

Mona phoned her friend who lives in another state. "How's it going, Nancy, taking care of Richard?"

"Oh, I'm hanging in there."

"Meaning . . . ?"

"Well, it's hard, you know."

"How is it hard?"

"Tell you the truth, I'm exhausted. But what can you do?"

"What *can* you do?"

"I'm doing everything, and I'm still falling behind."

"Nancy, have you thought about asking for help?"

"I don't need help. I can manage."

"No, you can't. Aren't you the one who just said, 'I'm falling behind'?"

"Hm. Yeah. I need help. It's time to ask."

Caregivers need their own caregivers, always.

CHAPTER 12

Suffering

Suffering is not the same as pain.

We recognize pain as an unpleasant sensation. Once we feel it, we can't help but think about it, and we routinely predict the worst scenario, a practice called "awfulizing." "Oh oh, my throat's sore. I'm going to miss that party." "This headache! My cancer's recurred." Such thoughts generate anxiety, depression, confusion, and anger, emotions that hurt on their own. Pain is what we feel, and suffering comes from what we make of the feeling.

Suffering is a normal phenomenon, and happens to be sickness' central feature. We seek medical help not because of some diagnosis, but because we're discomfited—perhaps by a pain, but at least as much by what the pain means to us, how the situation has affected us, affects us now, and might affect our future.

Recall when you were last sick, say with a severe cold. You felt under par, out of whack, and consequently maybe weak, useless, and ashamed of your dependency. Those feelings and the viral infection were related but separate entities. Sure, you looked forward to normal blood tests and other objective signs of improvement, but even more, you wanted to climb out of the dumps. You suffered from your cold, but more from your own self-generated sensations. *That is, your normal feelings in response to being sick were most of what actually distressed you.* It's curious, then, that biomedical practice views the alleviation of suffering as a tangential rather than essential goal.

We docs ought to ask patients, "What bothers you about being sick?" But we seldom ask it because it's a subjective question, we don't expect a useful answer from that realm, and it doesn't help us diagnose. Docs and patients alike popularly see suffering as generic, indistinguishable from person to person. So we address it uniformly, like smothering it beneath a blanket of drugs. That might make sense if suffering were indeed nonspecific, but it's not.

Suffering is unique to every individual and circumstance. People have told me their cancer made them feel depressed, frightened, useless, lonely, enraged, on and on. To appreciate that, try this experiment: ask sick friends how they are. Don't do it to out of courtesy or to fix them, only to honestly understand their suffering. Here's how that might go, condensed from conversations I had with my friend Steve over a period of two weeks:

"How are you doing?"

"Fine." (In Steve's case, that's F.I.N.E., for "Feelings I'm Not Expressing.")

"Can you tell me what bothers you about having cancer?"

"It means I'm going to die."

"Well . . . what bothers you about dying?"

"Are you kidding?"

"No, really. I'm serious."

He took a week to think about this, and said, "It's not about dying, I realized. Cancer's big, for sure, but what bothers me most now is what I'm missing."

"Like . . . ?"

"Well, at work we begin every morning with coffee and doughnuts, a half-hour of hanging out. The boss approves of it. I know it sounds kind of stupid, but for me that starts every day just right. Now, while I'm in treatment, I'm not working. Without my usual morning, my days feel directionless, like my life is over."

Had he failed to explore it, Steve's suffering would have remained unaddressably shapeless, but now he's identified at least one feature. He mentioned to a colleague how much he missed their ritual. Now, once a week, his office mates appear at his home early in the morning with coffee and doughnuts. Steve says, "My cancer isn't cured, but as trivial as it sounds, these sessions have restored some order and control, made me more comfortable."

Steve initiated this shift by examining his suffering instead of avoiding it. That's an uncommon act, since we assume only masochists would want to plunge into their angst. Since suffering by definition is unpleasant, we distract ourselves, deny it or repress it, maneuver around it any way we can. Avoidance works for the moment, but the suffering will persist inside us. When we finally decide to go intrepidly into its heart, we'll learn its details and then, like Steve, can act on them.

In addition to being distinctive, suffering is disorienting. Anatole Broyard (see page 64) wrote that his diagnosis of cancer was tantamount to being kidnapped across the border and abandoned in an alien land. He knew nothing of its geography, culture, or language, nor did he find allies there. His family and friends didn't "speak cancer." He'd never felt so lonely, helpless, and lost. I can't emphasize enough that it wasn't any tumor that kidnapped Broyard. His agonizing exile was his normal emotional response to simply learning his diagnosis.

If you've ever been told you had a serious illness such as cancer, you might recall that was the last word you heard in that conversation. You turned off as your world shattered. Gradually, as post-diagnosis numbness receded, tumultuous feelings roiled you: confusion, sadness, panic, and who knows what else. You thought, as many do, "Not only do I have cancer, but I'm losing my mind, too." No, you weren't. You were experiencing the anticipatable emotional uproar that decorates every serious diagnosis.

My medical training taught me that cancer is a tumor. That's like describing Hurricane Katrina as a summer rain. Far deeper and wider than we usually imagine, every serious illness is an entire circus of calamity, an explosion in the living room.

Especially in the case of cancer, suffering results partly from the paring away of what we think of as us. We can lose hair, organs, energy, fitness, appetite, sexuality, career, even friends. Our appearance can change almost daily, not unlike our bumpy ride through adolescence. This can shock our familiars and repulse those who are overcome by fear or who don't know what to say. Loss of our sense of stability can leave us unable to plan any kind of social life, which further isolates us. Suddenly shorn of our precious illusion of immortality, we feel estranged from those who still enjoy theirs.

One poignant example of loss involved Carl, who valued his work life so highly that absence from it to treat his prostate cancer fractured his sense of self. Call that strike one. Not only was he not working, a value in itself, but not bringing home the bacon, either, which equaled strike two. His treatment made him impotent and incontinent of urine, leaving him to feel his masculinity shredded: strike three. So it is that even though most men with prostate cancer won't die from it, they can be devastated nonetheless.

Suffering can take the form of guilt. When we're sick, we can feel at fault for our limitations. "I can't pick up the kids, Honey," you say. "You'll have to." Ashamed to depend on others, you say, "Thanks for offering, but I can manage." Aware that colleagues will have to take up your slack when you call in to work sick, you use your puniest, most apologetic voice.

It's especially easy to feel guilty when we believe we've caused our illness. For example, my friend Todd curses himself for his years of smoking. "I'm sure I brought on my lung cancer," he says. It makes no difference to him that not all smokers get cancer, and plenty of people who do get it never touched a cigarette. Whether Todd and others have actually created their illness is factually unanswerable. But torturing themselves about it only adds to their burden, so the issue begs therapeutic attention.

One of the more profound forms of suffering in illness is anxiety from losing certainty. Formerly black-and-white distinctions fade into shades of gray. Researching his illness, for example, Howard consulted an authoritative website that said some cases prove rapidly fatal, others vanish, and the rest fall in between. What, then, was he to conclude? When Marie asked if this new chemo would do the job, her doctor replied only that everyone's different. How is it that Jeanette felt okay while her blood test result was so haywire? Will Sarah's birthday be her last? Was Frank's wife withdrawn in order to give him privacy or because she was depressed?

Suffering is contagious, too. Everyone who associates with someone who's seriously ill suffers in their own way, and often more intensely. Looking at Ellen, you'd think it's her husband, Eric, not her, who's being treated for cancer. Ellen's side effects are minimal and her spirits buoyant, while Eric, continually seeking the elusive cure, is insomniac, anxious, and depressed.

So when you enter that sickroom, please don't focus on the patient alone. In each instance, look around and ask yourself, "Who's suffering here, now?" Maybe it's the patient's spouse or child. Maybe it's the nurse.

Maybe it's you.

CHAPTER 13

Treating Suffering

Much of what I've learned about addressing suffering came from an eight-hundred-year-old book, Dante's *Divine Comedy*. Since it was one of thirty assigned classics in a rushed college course, I came away with only a single but thankfully indelible memory: whatever it is that Dante does in hell, purgatory, and heaven, he's always accompanied by the Roman poet Virgil.

Dante tours this daunting landscape in its native vehicle, the emotional roller coaster. Witnessing Hell's literally diabolic tortures, he swings from denial to confusion to panic, but Virgil, always at his elbow, offers him the support needed in order to linger and learn. In our cancer center, we recommend that new patients find their Virgil as soon as is practical after diagnosis—a close friend, a cancer veteran, a professional counselor, or a support group.

Physicians increasingly recommend early counseling, too. Some prescribe tranquilizers or anti-depressants to mask unpleasant feelings—and occasionally they're temporarily needed—but these drugs bear the disadvantage of, well, masking feelings. They don't delete them, only Band-Aid them to stall their future emergence. As one of our support group members put it, "Buried feelings are buried alive." News of a serious diagnosis followed by hurried treatment, without time to process feelings (and hurry *is* sometimes appropriate), can result in Post-Traumatic Stress Disorder (PTSD) months later. To address these feelings whenever they emerge is to initiate healing.

Supported by your Virgil's guidance, you'll begin to comprehend the terrain of your suffering instead of resisting it, hellish though it may be. It'll gradually look more familiar and less alien and scary. Your emotions, huge and disturbing at first, will diminish, and eventually you'll find yourself still in the land of your illness, but shed of emotions: you don't feel great, you don't feel awful, simply present to the undeniable reality. This improves upon your previous whirlwind, and in happy addition, you'll feel calm enough to begin exploring this new place mindfully.

During the past century, as we were taught that advanced technology was the panacea that would render guides obsolete, physicians all but forgot how to accompany patients. So it is that today's Dantes too often wander through their Hell without Virgils.

Sensing that isolation as a need to fill, clever folks in high-tech thrall continually invent virtual Virgils. One example is computer softwares that ostensibly counsel. I consulted one, "Eliza" [1] which has been improved since her birth in the 1960s. You can visit her, too.

"Eliza, I was just diagnosed with cancer," I told her.

"I see," she said, then sunk into the anxiety-provoking silence some therapists use to prod their patients.

"It's serious. I could die."

"Do you believe it's normal to be sick, and you could die?"

"Well, I guess in a way it's normal, but it's scary."

"Come, come. Elucidate your thoughts."

"Wait a minute. I suspect you're a robot. How much is two plus two?"

"What answer would please you the most?"

At that point, I arose from the e-couch and bid Eliza farewell.

Of course, there are more advanced robots. The Panasonic Corporation recently announced it's developed one so effective that it's on order at dozens of hospitals. Imagine R2D2 turning up at your bedside. It doesn't look like a person except for the physician's face on the video screen, mounted where a head would be. The physician might not be in the hospital; she could be thousands of miles away. A camera in the robot transmits pictures of you to her. She operates controls to probe you here and there and maybe zoom in on a lesion. She offers you encouragement, texts orders to the nurses, and directs the robot to the next patient.

The robot might competently detect a complication or adjust your medication, but even the most sophisticated e-Virgil won't be able to alleviate your suffering since, like The Wizard of Oz's tin woodsman, it doesn't have a heart. The cleverest machine will inevitably lack compassion. It might claim it's compassionate, but then so do politicians.

Compassion means *suffering with*, attending so acutely to someone who's hurting that *we begin to feel their hurt*. Playing Virgil doesn't mean liking emotional pain, only feeling it. It's just a sensation, after all. (My first yoga teacher advised, "Don't think of it as pain; think of it as banana.") It's simply a feeling: the pain doesn't signify damage, and will ebb on its own. As a matter of fact, this sensation will persist to the extent we *avoid* feeling it.

Addressing suffering effectively is an obviously useful skill, since we're all certain to suffer. Sit down for this: we're going to lose everyone we love; either they'll die first or we will. Love and pain are so closely intertwined that avoiding one means avoiding the other as well, and what sort of life would that be? If you're not convinced, listen to more blues.

When I first tried on the Virgil role, facilitating cancer support groups, I was scared silly. What if a patient cried? Or lost control, or presented some problem I couldn't remedy? These worries sound neurotic now, but believe me, they can honestly distress a committed dispassionate scientist. To me, flagrant emotion was like a mirror to a vampire. Of course, people cried and lost control (including me), and I hardly ever encountered a problem I *could* fix. And much more. And I survived.

You—as a practitioner, relative, or friend of someone who's sick—might want to try playing Virgil. Here are a few guidelines from my previous book, *How to Heal* (Helios Press, 2003). I won't detail them here, but suffice it to say the effort requires your total attention.

- Tune in with your ears, eyes, and heart all at once.

- Sense the speaker's choice of words, metaphors, body language, and what's not said.

- Sense the feelings the message evokes in you.

- Do all this without planning what you'll say.

Surprise! You're engaging in intimate conversation. In doing this, I suggest you keep a couple of principles in mind. First, forget about the diagnosis, and second, don't try to fix.

Ignore the sickness's label. Whatever it is, the person has presumably hired competent practitioners to deal with it. For the purpose of alleviating suffering, the person, not the diagnosis, is of exclusive interest. If you think you're doing this work to influence the course of the physical illness, think otherwise: whatever the eventual outcome is, it will be ascribable to practically any cause. That is, your influence on the illness is permanently unknowable, so cluttering your mind with it will distract you from full attention to the person.

Don't try to fix suffering. While physical entities like a lawnmower or a damaged heart valve can possibly be fixed, suffering occupies a non-physical domain. No screwdriver can repair loneliness. Novelist Marcel Proust described the only effective strategy: "We are healed of suffering only by experiencing it to the full." That is, we get through it by getting through it, a process your help will accelerate.

Even knowing suffering can't be fixed, we try adamantly to fix it anyway, and inveterate caregivers like medical practitioners are especially adamant. We find ourselves saying things that sound hollow even in our own ears, like, "Don't worry about it" or, "It's going to be okay." That ploy is as common as it is useless, so it's worth asking why it persists. Even I, who can be apoplectic on the subject, find myself trying to fix.

Let's say you tell me, "I'm miserable. I can't keep food down, I hurt all over, I'm angry beyond belief, and it gets worse every day."

Where someone truly present might reply, "Tell me what's getting to you most," I sometimes find myself saying, "I know just the person you need to see." Or I'll say, "You need three grams of vitamin C daily." Or, "Oh, I felt like that once, and I got over it," or, "Read this," or, "Eat this." Those are fixes. Or call them "fixes," since I know in advance that you'll derive no benefit from them. I've had to ask myself why I, a well-meaning, well-informed, supposedly skilled person, would act this way.

It's not just me. It's most of us. Maybe we're hard-wired that way. If you've read the Old Testament's *Book of Job* (I recommend the modern American English translation by Stephen Mitchell, HarperCollins Publishers, 1992), you'll see that my lame suggestions resemble what Job's friends offered him: I know why you're suffering and what you need to do about it. They probably realized as they spoke that they were blowing hot air, too.

Here's what I've discovered: *I offer fixes when I am suffering.* I suffer because compassion hurts. After all, I'm essentially saying to you, "Tell me how you're suffering until I feel it." I actually want to feel it, but I can take only so much pain, and then my insides rebel and scream "Enough!"

It would be unseemly, though, to tap my wristwatch and say, "Whoa, gotta move on. Where does the time go?" So instead I say, "I'll give you this clinic's website" or, "I heard about a promising clinical trial in Albuquerque." Sure enough, my fix flash-freezes your narrative. I've accomplished my purpose, which was to end *my* suffering.

Any caregiver's prime tool is caring for oneself. To paraphrase philosopher Alan Watts, we should be in the suffering but not of the suffering, performing a kind of aikido that lets others' feelings touch us as they pass through us. One model toward that end is the Tibetan Buddhist *tong len*, a breathing practice in which one visualizes inhaling suffering and exhaling happiness to all beings. I breathe in your pain and breathe it out. Sometimes this is all that's needed. In Tibet or anywhere else, witnessing grief seems to cut it in half. Obviously, this sort of caregiving is not the spiritual hemorrhage our culture usually practices. Here both parties come away feeling better. That sounds like healing to me.

CHAPTER 14

Community as Medicine

Thirty years ago I worked for an agency for disabled people. Funded by a grant, we enrolled forty clients into our common human experiences, including relationships, work, expression, disability, spirituality, and death and dying. In other words, we chatted about our lives. (I was surprised, by the way, to hear more than one member remark, "I didn't know you could talk about this stuff.")

We believed that in some way these meetings might influence participants' health, so we recorded their healthcare use before and after the project, and again six months later. Following these meetings, their medical visits dropped 40 percent and held there. When we reported our findings to grant agency officers, they didn't believe us, and declined to renew our funding.

Today our discovery would be back-page news. An article in the *New Yorker* in 2011, written by writer/surgeon Atul Gawande, related studies indicating that community is a medicine as potent as any pill or surgery. To begin, Gawande points out that a small fraction of patients uses a grossly disproportionate share of healthcare. For example, 1 percent of the Camden, New Jersey, population accounts for *30 percent* of the city's total medical expense. That 1 percent isn't scattered randomly, but clustered in low-income neighborhoods, housing projects, nursing homes, and assisted living facilities. Researchers call these foci of overuse "hotspots."

This fits with what we already know about those who live in hotspots. Most are too poor to pay for healthcare, nor can they find a doctor who accepts Medicaid (publicly funded health insurance for low-income people, which remunerates docs triflingly), so they go to the nearest emergency department (ED). Some, unable to afford bus fare, summon ambulances. While most of these patients are present with non-emergencies—colds, flu, rashes—they generate inordinate cost, since EDs, which must maintain hyper-trained staff and expensive equipment, must also treat all patients regardless of ability to pay. Hospitals try to recoup these losses by overcharging elsewhere in their system, calling the practice "cost averaging." Patients who have money or insurance, then, ultimately pay for unnecessarily expensive care of the poor.

Gawande describes a number of features of the Affordable Care Act ("Obamacare") that aim to address ED overuse and to lower healthcare costs in general. He writes,

> The new health-reform law . . . authorizes new forms of Medicare and Medicaid payment to encourage the development of "medical homes" and "accountable care organizations"—doctors' offices and medical systems that get financial benefits for being more accessible to patients, better organized, and accountable for reducing the over-all costs of care.

Thus publicly funded low-tech care centers have opened inside some housing projects and nursing homes. Practitioners and trained volunteers visit patients where they live. Some programs offer classes, and even organize and advocate for residents. And it seems to work: these strategies reduce medical visits by . . . you guessed it, 40 percent.

I imagine this approach is successful because sometimes what people actually need is only a little education, encouragement, or social contact. When I practiced emergency medicine, it seemed to me and to colleagues that many of our patients were simply miserable, and sought medical help because their despair was emerging through their physiology. Psychologists know that one antidote for psychological pain is physical pain, which can eventually present as physical illness. It's a condition getting known in medical circles as "terribly-sad-life syndrome."[1]

I saw a milder version of this when a man in his late twenties appeared in our emergency department at two o'clock one morning, complaining of a "grating" belly pain. Since no other patients were waiting at that hour, I asked him about his life. He was employed at a local auto assembly plant. He described his job, which he called "the daily grind." His boss was an "abrasive" man who was "wearing me down." My hearing perked up at the consistent metaphors, but I had no idea of their significance. He finally paused, looked into the distance, and said, "I wonder if I'm talking about my pain or my job." Suddenly that statement made sense in a strange way. But unfamiliar with this mode of seeing, I said nothing and simply arranged for tests and a clinic appointment. We never saw him again. Six months later, though, we received a post card in which he said he'd quit his job, moved to another city, started his own business, and his belly had stopped hurting.

I did nothing for this man but hear him out. He could have spoken to anyone, but chose me even though I was unaccustomed to viewing symptoms through an existential lens. If he'd felt safe speaking to, say, a friend, he might have come to the same conclusion. More importantly, he might have learned from this experience to see other problems in his life as not medical but social. In the event, he and I were two unwitting members of a small healing community.

That term, "healing community," is redundant. Mindfully being with others is itself therapeutic. A study of seven thousand men and women found that people unconnected to others were three times as likely to die over the course of nine years as those who had strong social ties.

That study inventoried lifestyles, too. As you might guess, the people with fewest ties and unhealthiest styles died soonest, and those who lived healthfully and had strong social ties lived longest. But—wrap your mind around this—those with close social ties and *unhealthy* lifestyles actually lived longer than their more health-promoting but less connected counterparts.

It's reasonable, then, to wonder whether self-centeredness is a health risk. Researchers recorded the conversations of nearly six hundred men, of whom a third had heart disease. They found that those who used first-person singular pronouns most often—I, me, mine—were likeliest to have heart disease and most susceptible to heart attacks.

In another study of over two thousand men who'd had heart attacks, survival was more closely associated with social connectedness than the heart drug being tested.

A study of women with breast cancer found that the length of their survival, all else equal, was proportional to the number of their "confidants," defined as sharers of personal secrets. Those with no confidants survived the shortest time; those with six confidants—the maximum number the study tracked—survived the longest.

If I suffer an incurable illness, I'll benefit from optimum medical care and also from contact with others, especially learning from veteran patients how to accommodate to my condition. Joan, a woman recently diagnosed with lung cancer, attended her first meeting of our support group. She expressed the doleful notion, common a generation ago, that a cancer diagnosis means imminent doom. But here she met Ann, who's lived with metastatic lung cancer for twenty-two years. Having now witnessed wider possibilities, Joan left the meeting obviously more buoyant.

If I suffer an illness that results from lifestyle, I can learn how others in like situations altered their habits, and gain enough support to attempt a similar course. Milt is a middle-aged bachelor whose job requires him to sit at a computer forty hours weekly. Jack, a few desks away, commented to him that he was looking alarmingly out of shape.

Milt said, "Well, you look like you're pretty fit. How do you do it?"

"A year ago I felt so sluggish I was starting to get depressed. So I joined a club, and I work out every day."

"I tried a club," said Milt. "It's pretty boring."

"It is. But it's a great place to meet new people, and it's given me a social life again. Maybe that's really why I go there."

Soon after Milt joined Jack at the club, he met Virginia, whose friend had recently persuaded her to join. Now Milt and Virginia regularly exercise together, and a careful observer might note an early six-pack in Milt's abs.

Social contact isn't just physically therapeutic. It's a vitamin for mental health, too. Most conversations boil down to, "I'll tell you my experiences and what I made of them, and you tell me yours." Psychologists call this process "reality testing." Born ignorant of the world, we gradually learn how to navigate with the help of lessons from our relatives, friends, and the wider culture. Comparing my sense of things with others' versions, I'll see that some people have crafted more graceful paths than others. Maybe I'll learn I've behaved in ways healthier people do not, such as being more competitive than necessary, flying off the handle inappropriately, accepting abuse, or withholding love. And maybe others will find in me some quality to emulate or avoid. We all do this to some degree; in aggregate, it's what we call civilization.

But civilization as we know it might be an endangered species, as an array of new and seductive technologies invites us to separate. The October 2010 *New Yorker* cover depicted parents chaperoning their trick-or-treating kids around a neighborhood. Each adult face is lit by the blue glow of a cell phone. Until recently I wouldn't have imagined such a rupture of the familial bond. But today a staggering number of us walk the streets looking not into the eyes of our kids or of others, but down, into our own palms.

I recently noticed a friend at the local farmer's market but didn't approach her since she was on her cell phone. I wanted to ask her something like, "Why on this perfect day, amidst a display of the finest foods in the state and in the presence of dozens of your friends, do you prefer the cyberworld? What in that phone could possibly attract you more than what's here now?"

Conversely, I could have asked, "Why, when you obviously want to be on your phone, are you here in this busy *mercado* instead of in a quiet place, focusing your attention on the person you're speaking with?"

I imagine her answer to either question would be, "I'm multitasking."

Apparently not content to fill our waking hours with busyness, we've up-shifted to double-timing. As we watch *Dancing With the Stars* on our smartphones, we simultaneously read a webpage decrying multitasking's notorious inefficiency. My friend might believe she's at the market and communicating with a friend, but she's actually half-engaged with and half-withdrawn from each. As the 1970s radio comedy group Firesign Theater sang, "How can you be in two places at once when you're nowhere at all?"

Social withdrawal has become so pervasive that community is at risk of joining the long-playing record and dial telephone in history's dustbin. Instead of chatting with neighbors on the front steps or attending the grange dance, we collapse onto the couch for another numbing tube dose. We're retreating in large numbers into the virtual cocoons of home theaters, gated neighborhoods, corporate malls, and dark-windowed SUVs. Online social networks offer an illusion of community in the same way junk foods pretend nutrition. Proud to have collected hundreds of "friends," we text and tweet in solitude. As a popular calypso song puts it,

"I journey to me local coffee house
to sip a cup and socialize
All of de tables are occupied by
elegant gals and guys
But nobody say a single word,
dey be staring at dere laptop screens
Wid all of dis classy company,
dey prefer to talk to machines
Dey be zombies, zombies, passing as one of us . . ."

Self-absorption, when florid, is considered a mental illness, Narcissistic Personality Disorder (diagnosis code 301.81 in psychiatry's bible, the *Diagnostic and Statistical Manual of Mental Disorders*, or "DSM"). The psychiatrists who fashioned the DSM's current fifth edition battled for years over whether to keep or delete narcissism. Is it a mental illness, to remain in the manual, or is it so common now as to be arguably normal? In a split decision, the editors voted to keep it a diagnosis, but let's see if it's retained in DSM-6.

Mental health will benefit to the extent we maintain community, stay in real-life, real-time contact with one another. Please think about that and text me your ideas, and while you're at it, send me a selfie.

CHAPTER 15

The Embodied Mind

Explaining emotions, my neurology professor said, "It's only your dopamine talking."

He meant that the mind is essentially an illusion created by neurotransmitters in the brain: consciousness is a product of chemistry. Doing its best to ignore human subjectivity, biomedicine conceives the mind as an illusion created by molecular reactions.

That seems sensible enough, after all. We take a mind-altering drug, and sure enough, our mind gets altered. Push this concept to its limit, though, and the free will, humor, and passion we believe we enjoy—in fact, the very sensation of enjoyment, the juice of life—is nothing more than chemical puppetry.

Curiously, this view, however hardcore conventional, has never been proven. The truth might actually be the opposite, that consciousness causes chemical changes in the brain. Easy cases can be made: when you think about someone you love, your pituitary gland releases euphoria-conferring endorphins. Psychologist Robert Ornstein wrote in his 1977 book *The Psychology of Consciousness* that he'd intended to explain the chemical basis of consciousness, but was surprised to find he'd described instead the consciousness basis of brain chemistry.

While consciousness and chemistry evidently play both directions, biomedicine, insisting on the primacy of the physical body, relegates the mind to a separate, secondary status.

So it is that physicians distinguish between physical, "organic" illnesses and "functional" ones, mental events. An illness qualifies as organic when a change in structure or chemistry can be observed. The pus on tonsils, the elevated blood glucose level, or the tumor noted on an MRI are unquestionably real.

A functional illness, on the other hand, isn't as "real," since no structural or chemical changes can be found to account for the patient's symptoms. Say you experience memory loss, exhaustion, insomnia, and other discomforts. You go from doctor to chiropractor to psychologist, and everyone throws up their hands. Finally a naturopath diagnoses chronic fatigue syndrome.

"At last!" you exclaim. But then you learn that treatments seem hit-and-miss, and your medical doctor doesn't even believe such a disorder exists. You're left feeling confused, abandoned, and less confident in medical science. Other diagnoses in this misty realm include, depending on whom you ask, fibromyalgia, multiple environmental sensitivity, *candida* allergy, ADD, ileocecal valve disorder, seasonal affective disorder, social anxiety disorder, sex addiction, and others we'll no doubt hear about next month.

If "functional" gets pinned on you, you'll likely take it to mean it's psychosomatic, it's all in your head, it's imaginary, you need to see a shrink, or you're a hypochondriac, malingerer, or outright fake, none of which feels like a proper fit. Functional illness frustrates doctors as well as patients. Whether a given disorder is "real" or "not real," these people are suffering, and if I as a physician haven't been trained to treat their emotions, I can only hammer away with my usual pills and surgeries, or refer them to my least favorite specialist.

Were we to view people through a lens that integrates body and mind rather than one that values the body over its alleged mental by-product, we'd no longer need to agonize about what is and isn't real. In addition, we'd gain insights into where illness can originate. So here's an integrating attempt: *when you look at someone's body, you're seeing their mind in action.*

If you're familiar with "body language," you know my wink is more than an eyelid flutter. It's a message, even if I'm not aware of its content and even if I don't know I winked. If the past century of psychology taught us anything, it's that human behavior is meaningful, however unconsciously so. Hardly any gesture is accidental. My grimace says something, as does the tilt of my eyebrow and my crossed legs.

We can't stop expressing. Recall how carefully you'd arranged yourself on that first date. Clothing covers us and at the same time constitutes a carefully crafted message. Ornamentation—hair, jewelry, tattoos—speaks volumes. Our vocal tone communicates as much as the words it shapes. We emit sweat and pheromones and who knows what else. Some people claim the ability to smell fear and lust.

In fact, where do we not leave evidence? From every pore we broadcast the meanings we make of the world. Words can lie, but the organ of behavior, the body, can't. It can't shut up, either. As dancer Martha Graham put it, "Movement is the barometer telling the state of the soul's weather."

Through repetition, our conduct affects our very shape. The bowling arm grows larger than its mate. Hikers' leg muscles expand, and those who no longer walk see their legs wither. Slouch through your adolescence, and like your mother warned, that posture may become permanent. Mark Twain observed, "After the age of thirty, you're responsible for your face." The medical word for body shape, *habitus*, seems a curious choice . . . until we explore the body-mind in action, and realize shape is in appreciable degree the crystallization of habit.

We receive information, too, as abundantly as we transmit it. In fact, we absorb so much more sense data than we can consciously process that attending to all of it would overwhelm us. High-speed films, shot at thousands of frames per second and then shown in real time, reveal mothers and their babies mutually mimicking faster than the eye can see. During a few milliseconds, the mom grimaces and the baby copies. One coos and instantly the other echoes. Ask the mom what she's doing, and she'll relate only what she's aware of, playing with her baby, but at a deeper level, she and the baby are bouncing expressions back and forth to literally learn each other. Part of psychotherapy training is practice in slowing such "films" in order to become more sensitive to the massive spray of information coming from clients.

In addition to sending and receiving information, our bodies accumulate it. When I first began practicing yoga a half-life ago, I was chagrined to find myself inexplicably emotional in certain poses. I'd giggle uncontrollably in backbends, get lightheaded and fall over in some standing poses, and come close to tears in even gentle forward bends. My teacher explained, "Oh, you didn't know? Muscles store emotions without us being aware of it, and when we put our attention into those areas the feeling can flood out. No big deal. Just put up with it, and it'll stop." He was right; the outbursts gradually disappeared. I've heard from massage practitioners, too, that often, as their fingers awaken regions held numb for years, clients experience sudden catharsis.

One way of seeing the body-mind, then, is as a fleshy antenna, continually receiving, transmitting, and storing information.

This model shouldn't seem impractically strange, as we already read body language routinely. For example, consider mundane exchanges like this:

"So what did he say?"

"He didn't say much at all. It was that smile and the look he gave me."

"And like you mentioned, his after-shave and manicure . . ."

Once we accept that each of us comprises a unique inner of meaning, we can no longer see ourselves as interchangeable "consumers" and "providers" of healthcare. Visualizing himself in that wider perspective, author Anatole Broyard (see p. 64) wrote, "My ideal doctor would 'read' my poetry. Inside every patient, there's a poet trying to get out."

If you've ever wondered whether your illness was somehow connected to the way you lead your life, consider that meaningful behavior doesn't stop at the social level. It extends into physiology. Why would we want to believe, for example, that a frown is a message, but a quickened heartbeat must be random? If slumping can signify depression, why can't plummeted resistance announce overwhelming stress?

Plenty of evidence indicates the mind's influence in pathogenesis, the initiation of illness. In her book *Sleep Paralysis: Night-mares, Nocebos, and the Mind-Body Connection*, medical anthropologist Shelley Adler describes the death, in their sleep, of one hundred seventeen Hmong men who'd immigrated to the United States. They were posthumously diagnosed with "Sudden Unexpected Nocturnal Death Syndrome," or SUNDS (hardly a diagnosis, actually, since it means these people suddenly died at night and we don't know why). Adler concludes,

> It is my contention that in the context of severe and ongoing stress related to cultural disruption and national resettlement (exacerbated by intense feelings of powerlessness about existence in the United States), and from the perspective of a belief system in which evil spirits have the power to kill men who do not fulfill their religious obligations, the solitary Hmong man confronted by the numinous terror of the night-mare (and aware of its murderous intent) can die of SUNDS.

Doctors guess that the physiologic culprit behind SUNDS is a cardiac arrhythmia. Perhaps that's so, but the question remains: *why* does a heart go amok, and why in this person, at this time? Do cardiologists ask themselves if these scores of men lived with troubled hearts? SUNDS brings to mind similar mysterious lethalities around the world, especially in Asia. In the Philippines it's called *bangungot*. It's *pokkuri* in Japan, *dab tsog* in Laos, and *lai tai* in Thailand. In Haiti it's ascribed to voodoo. A phenomenon this widespread is worth considering not as some rogue supernatural visitation, but as further evidence that the human mind thoroughly informs the body.

Of course, illness-as-poetry is far from biomedicine's view. In a hospital corridor I asked a cardiologist friend, "Tell me, do you ever think of your patients as heavy-hearted? Stone-hearted? Heartbroken? That sort of thing?"

"Sure, my patients go through the same kind of life hassles everyone does."

"What I mean is: do you think they might be telling a single story, not two? That their cardiomyopathy might express that they've been too big-hearted or soft-hearted, or that their angina is heartache from a major loss?"

"Can we talk about this later? I need to go put a stent in."

I should have asked my question over a beer, not in a biomedical temple. You don't ask a monsignor to ponder Confucianism beneath St. Peter's dome.

Since biomedicine understands patients strictly as physical entities, a shift in someone's physiology looks abnormal—a syndrome in search of a name—rather than a normal response to some experience. Though any nine-year-old knows blushing expresses embarrassment, I once heard a colleague call it a "dysautonomia." This bias tends to medicalize much of human behavior, defining it as suitable for treatment. Seen through such a filter, a rise in my blood pressure after a nasty stranger accosts me means I'm afflicted with RMH, Rudeness-Mediated Hypertension. Or after my boss reviles me daily for twenty-four years, such that now I find my neck permanently withdrawn, turtle-like, into my chest,

I'm a hapless victim of the dreaded SNS, Short Neck Syndrome. I wax facetious here to illuminate a serious disconnect. If we were to address traffic accidents the way biomedicine views human beings, we'd scrutinize every car part while hardly glancing at the drivers.

We are hard put not to admit that experience can alter physiology. A landmark study done by Kaiser Permanente in San Diego [1] demonstrated how closely adverse childhood experiences ("ACEs") correlate with health problems in adulthood. Some seventeen thousand people, average age fifty-seven, three-quarters of them college-educated, were interviewed in detail about their childhoods. They were asked specifically about ACEs, including emotional, physical, and sexual abuse, household dysfunction like family violence, alcoholism, imprisonment, and mental illness, and emotional and physical neglect. Researchers assigned patients a point for every ACE in their history, and then tracked them over the next fourteen years for medical visits, hospitalizations, drug use, death, and other factors.

High ACE scores correlated perfectly with increased incidence in adulthood of memory impairment, cigarette use, drug and alcohol abuse, liver and lung disease, depression, suicide, number of prescriptions filled, and, fascinatingly, number of unexplainable symptoms. The study is being continued, and will probably last until all subjects have died. At this point there haven't been enough deaths to know whether high ACE scores are associated with shorter lives, but the patients in the study who've lived longest have the lowest ACE scores.

In another study exploring the link between experience and illness, Australian researchers found that women who were raped or sexually abused tend to suffer a lifetime of mental disorder, including impaired quality of life, overall disability, and increased suicide attempts.

In another study, the American Psychological Association found that a positive social atmosphere in the workplace confers longevity. Employees who enjoyed collegial support and positive social interactions were less likely to die over a twenty-year period than those who reported a less friendly work environment.

Maybe such revelations aren't surprising, as you already suspected that traumas can cultivate sickness, and that happy people live longer. None of this is news to the attentive, yet when we or someone close to us falls ill, we tend to overlook these principles and default to the more popular view, that the illness resulted from pure chance, so all that's called for is standard biomedical remedy.

I saw a man who complained of agonizing sciatic pain, which he described as "shocks from my back down my legs, like I'm in an electric chair." He told me he'd lost three successive wives to breast cancer. "I worry that in some magical way I was responsible even though I know that's not so," he said. "It's crazy. But I'm afraid to get involved again. I can't help but feel like I'm carrying some curse."

I asked what I felt was an obvious question. "Have you wondered whether your feeling about your wives' illnesses might somehow be connected with your back pain?"

He got angry. "Of course not! I have a pile of MRIs that show displaced discs all over my spine. No, this is *real!*"

He went on to have surgery—his fourth—that left him in exactly the same condition. To him, a "real" disorder required "real" treatment. Spinal surgery is a daunting proposition for anyone, but to him it was probably less threatening than unpacking his emotional baggage.

That's a common conflict. When we fall ill, we sometimes speculate on whether our condition reflects some issue in our life, but then drop it like a hot coal when the answer looks positive. The message might be, "Yes, there is something amiss, and honestly facing it is certain to eventuate in change. Now, would you rather proceed into change's *terra incognita*, or settle for what you live with now?" Absent guidance or support for the intimidating journey, we usually choose the pill rather than life review. Imagine the possibilities, though, if we healthcare practitioners, attending to patients' minds as skillfully as we do their bodies, were to apply our technologic Band-Aids *and* encourage them to embark on their healing adventures.

CHAPTER 16

The *D* Word

W e don't like death.

I was at a hot springs last year, soaking alone at dawn, contemplating my eventual demise. As I wondered how the world could possibly limp on without me, a fellow in a ten-gallon hat swaggered onto the deck and called, "How you doing?" Unwilling to compromise my silence, I smiled and nodded.

"Hot in there?"

"Sorry," I said, "but I'm here on a retreat. I'd rather not talk."

He held up his palms. "Oh! Excuse me. Don't want to intrude . . . What do you mean 'retreat?'"

I realized nothing short of playing the D card would work. I was truthful. Speaking for all of us, I said, "Well, I have a terminal condition. I'm going to die."

He blanched and backed out, too unnerved to inquire further.

That *D* word unglues many of us. Do we avoid talking about death because it's scary, or is it scary because we don't talk about it? Ask people to name their greatest fear, and most will say "the unknown," of which death is the paramount example. Fearing it, we hide it away and so fear it all the more. What would an alien anthropologist say about a society that maintains such a cycle?

Influenced by death's understandably negative reputation, some doctors unconsciously curtail their approach to seriously ill patients. A woman with pancreatic cancer said, "I asked my oncologist whether my anemia is from my cancer or the chemo. He just looked at me and walked out. It's not that he isn't communicative. I overheard him talking with another patient right before he saw me. He answered her questions about lymphoma just fine."

I said, "Why do you think he behaved differently with you?"

"Well, as far as I know, her prognosis is much better than mine."

"Meaning . . ."

"Well, I think he's kind of given up on me. It seemed it didn't matter what the answer to my question is since I won't be here long, anyway. I'm Dead Woman Walking."

I suspect she's right, especially since I remember acting many years ago like her doctor did. I subtly avoided patients I considered doomed. I doubt this woman's doctor is aware he did that, but she's made an appointment to talk with him about it, and I believe he's educable.

One reason doctors too seldom discuss end-of-life issues with patients and their families is that they don't get paid for it. And that's so because the greater society feels the subject, ostensibly morbid and scary, is an inappropriate departure from biomedicine's salvation mission. So it is that American docs earn thousands for a brain operation, but not a cent for helping guide people through their darkest hour. A provision in an early version of the Affordable Care Act of 2010 ("Obamacare") specified paying doctors to hold such conversations, but no sooner was this made public than millions interpreted it as "death panels" intent on pulling Grandma's plug, and the provision was dropped.

If one way we dodge the Reaper is by denying his presence, another is by spinning wishful fairy tales that glorify healthcare's capabilities. We attribute resurrective power to physicians, many of who, reluctant to crush that flattering illusion, do anything they can to prolong life. At some point, though, the added quantity of life costs the balance of its quality, and the noble attempt decays into prolongation of suffering.

We know that simply talking in advance about death and dying delivers substantial benefits. In a recent study, over six hundred advanced-cancer patients were asked whether they'd had end-of-life conversations with their physicians. Those who had experienced an average 36 percent lower medical expense, as most chose to rule out various high-tech interventions. (This is no small savings, as Medicare, the government medical insurance for seniors, spends nearly 30 percent of its budget in beneficiaries' final year of life.) The study concluded that higher costs—typically the result of more intensive care—were associated with a *worse* quality of life during patients' final week . . . and in addition, they didn't extend lives anyway.

End-of-life conversations should generate "advance directives," as they're known, legal orders regarding your medical treatment should you be unable to direct care yourself. One example, the "Durable Power of Attorney for Healthcare," or DPAHC, simply asks you to specify an agent to make decisions for you if you can't. The form is available through most hospices and even stationery stores, and doesn't require an attorney's help.

If you create your own advance directives, be aware that when these documents are needed, they often can't be found, having been filed away with old receipts or wadded up in a glove compartment. Without your document, you'll be subject to a hospital's default policy, which might be antithetical to your wishes. So make a half-dozen copies. Give one to your specified agent. Have one placed in your medical file. If you're hospitalized, be sure one's added to your chart.

While some feel that preparing advance directives is a dark task, the process actually offered me revelations about my life. When I created my own DPAHC, I named my wife as my agent. Knowing me better than anyone else, Ronnie is most likely to make decisions I'd have made. But, I worried, what if she didn't?

I imagined myself in an ICU, apparently comatose but still able to hear and understand. My doctors ask her what she'd like them to do. I hear her answer them, and I think: uh oh, exactly wrong. That's not at all what I'd like. But I can't speak. I'm at the mercy of her decision. I fall into an emotional tailspin. On the way down, I meet a thought coming up: haven't I learned over past decades that sometimes I'm wrong and she's right? Why am I sure she's wrong now? If I really meant my marriage vows, don't I literally trust her with my life? I finally surrender when I realize my only other choice is to fruitlessly torture myself.

In life's home stretch, where illness, disability, and death are ever more likely, acceptance begins to look like a terrifically useful tool. Not at all the same as doing nothing, acceptance requires great strength of will. In my experience, cancer support group participants almost unanimously take exception to the newspaper obituaries eulogizing someone who "lost her valiant battle against cancer."

"I'm not fighting anything," said one. "I'm just trying to live with the damn disease."

Living with it includes living with its treatments. We can't but notice that as time passes and interventions accumulate, our life is less composed of joy and more of preservation. At that point, the "quantity-versus-quality" dilemma has arisen, and we have serious decisions to make. Our question might be, "Is my treatment helping me more than it's hurting me?" or, put literarily, "Is the game worth the candle?" While this issue arises regularly in real life, it's hardly ever discussed publicly, which is one reason conventional wisdom conceives no alternative to nonstop treatment.

Daisy announced to her cancer support group, "I just found out my cancer is stage four now. Surgery's out of the question, and I've had it with chemo and radiation. I can't ignore the handwriting on the wall anymore. So I've decided to live out the rest of my life with only comfort care."

Her comment split the group into two camps. One member, Art, pleaded, "But you have to do something about the cancer."

Esther, another member, said, "No you don't. I completely support you, Daisy. Enough is enough."

Daisy replied, "Yeah, that's pretty much the way my friends took my decision. Some thought I'd done right, others were appalled. Most of my family said I was crazy for not going for more treatment. I can understand that, but I told them as gently as possible, 'Look, it's my body, my life, and I have to do what I have to do.'"

Daisy described how she arrived at her decision. "Early on, during my first chemo sessions, I asked my doctor what would happen if these medications became ineffective.

"'Not to worry,' he told me. 'If this regimen fails, I have a whole shelf of others.'

"Well, that made sense. But since then I've been through the whole shelf, and lived with a shelf of side effects. Cancer's a big disease, so needs big treatment. I get that. The medical people do what they can for the diarrhea, the mouth sores, the neuropathies and so on. But it's hard to live with all of them, not to mention the fatigue, 'chemo brain,' and especially the lifestyle, if you can call it that: I'm spending more and more of my time in medical settings.

"Here's what it comes down to: the more treatment I get, the less life there is for me to live. For hours every day I'm either getting examined or tested or treated, or pleading on the phone with insurance androids. My time with my family is almost nil, and doing anything outside my home is close to unimaginable. My life's essentially become trying to stay alive. I don't want to hate the rest of it. I hear about this strategy's ultimate extent—patients kept artificially going just for the sake of being alive. That doesn't sound attractive to me. No, thanks."

Daisy persuaded her doctor to refer her to hospice, where she was assured she'd be optimally comforted. Still, she says,

"When I see my doctor, he kind of shakes his head, like he wants to say, 'Daisy, you quit too soon.' I don't think he realizes that his discomfort is his, not mine. I wrote him a letter asking for an appointment just to talk because I want him fully on board."

Daisy showed me the letter. Part of it reads, "I come from a place between two mighty rivers, the Mississippi and the Missouri. They flood, and I've done my share of filling and carrying sandbags, and cleaning up. In the end, though, the rivers take everything . . ."

The palliation Daisy receives is light years beyond that of a few decades ago. In 1962, when my aunt Gertie was suffering advanced cancer, she was operated on twice. I now recognize those procedures as senseless, and served only to treat her doctor's anxiety. He finally shifted her to palliative care, which was rudimentary then, consisting mainly of hydration. Painkillers were withheld from fear she might "get addicted."

Even a generation after Gertie died, the highly respected "S.U.P.P.O.R.T." study,[1] published in 1995, revealed that dying people's care wishes were seldom discussed, let alone honored. Fewer than half of physicians knew whether their patients wished to avoid cardiopulmonary resuscitation. Half of do-not-resuscitate (DNR) orders were written within two days of death, signifying that conversation on the subject had been postponed until the situation was starkly undeniable. Palliation meant minimal and often inadequate treatment: half the conscious patients who died in the hospital reported moderate to severe pain at least half the time. That is, practitioners recognized the approaching end of life yet still under-treated dying patients' suffering.

Today, hospices around the country offer nursing visits, counseling, expert pain control, caregiver respite, and other services. You're eligible for most hospices when your physician certifies you'll likely die within six months. (Of course, some patients outlive that prediction.)

Insurance carriers that cover this care generally pay only if palliation is the sole intervention. In other words, as a hospice patient, you can't be treated for the illness itself; you can only receive symptomatic "comfort" care. Though this makes some sense, it gets tricky when illness treatment happens also to be palliative. For example, you might be surprised, as I was, to learn that sometimes chemotherapy agents are more effective than opiates in controlling cancer pain.

Hospices constantly lament that families are often referred too late—sometimes within days of death—for routines and relationships to effectively establish themselves. This is sad but understandable considering prevalent views. Hospice intervention, with its message that death is ever closer, can fracture the protective denial of decline. In addition, doctors may fear loss of some treatment they feel is essential, or that hospice referral might connote medical failure.

If, as it's said, the Reaper always bats last, then "medical failure," if you want to call it that, is ultimately inevitable. That contradicts the popular fantasy of medicine's omnipotence, so hospice referral can seem to patients like their doctor has given up, handed them their pink slip, all but evicted them from the company of the breathing. When life and death are considered opposites, regular medical care means living, and hospice care, dying.

Yet they aren't opposites. Since birth entails eventual death without exception, living and dying are aspects of a single process. In fact, dying occurs throughout life, as we replace most of our cellular structure every seven years or so. With later cycles, the replacements are smaller, less efficient, and, we must admit, less attractive. If we are dying a bit even as we live, if death is actually a lifelong stowaway . . .

. . . *why not palliate everyone?*

Why not support all patients like we do the "dying" so well today? Why not provide expert pain coverage and counseling along with standard medical intervention in every instance? Why not, as Dr. Trudeau advised a century ago, "comfort always?" Ironically, I look forward to the day when hospices are no longer necessary because palliation is integral to all healthcare.

This isn't such a pipe dream, as doctors already palliate more than they know.

"I've been treating this seventy-year-old woman for emphysema," a doctor friend told me. "She's on some meds, plus oxygen at home. She's smoked a couple of packs a day for the past fifty years, and she's not about to quit. She takes a drag from her cigarette, then one from her oxygen tank, back and forth. I'm tempted to fire her. I mean, this is absurd. I like her plenty, but she claws back any advantage I can give her. What do you think I should do?"

I've learned to answer tough questions by asking another. "Well, you've thought of firing her. Why haven't you?"

"I'd feel awful. Whatever she's doing, she's still my patient."

"What does that mean to you—that she's your patient?"

"Despite my complaints, I really like her, and I'll stand by her no matter what. But this is beyond what I was trained in, diagnosis and treatment. I try to be nice to her. I hug her every visit, I sit close, pat her on the shoulder, listen to all her stories. In fact, all I can do is listen, since I can't offer much other treatment. But I'm not a hospice doctor. I don't do palliative."

"You don't?"

I like to think of him and similar-minded colleagues as palliating not only their patients, but moribund American healthcare itself by offering closer personal contact *along with* appropriate medical treatment. This new bedside manner will grow and spread as we revisit our concepts of health and illness, diagnosis and treatment, the patient-doctor and body-mind relationships, apportionment of responsibility, what we want from healthcare versus what we need, and what we're prepared to provide one another. That will require time and effort, but given the present system's rate of descent, there's no other choice.

CHAPTER 17

Obamacare:
A Half-Stepping Stone

The Affordable Care Act of 2010 is an attempt to fix our fragmented, cumbersome, and inequitable healthcare system. Bearing obvious benefits along with limitations, it's a half-step in the right direction. It covers millions of Americans previously uncovered. It offers expanded no-cost preventive care, including immunizations, diabetes, and cancer screenings, and counseling for smoking and alcohol abuse. It funds research seeking more cost-efficient means of healthcare. There are no annual or lifetime dollar limits on essential benefits. Children can stay on their parents' plan until they turn twenty-six. No one can be denied coverage because of a pre-existing medical problem. And federal financial assistance is available to help pay medical insurance premiums or out-of-pocket expenses for those below certain income levels.

On the other hand, some ACA coverage will be skimpy and unaffordable, and thirty-one million Americans will remain uncovered (including five million because some governors have opted out of Medicaid).[1] Concludes Harvard public health professor Dr. Steffie Woolhandler, "Obamacare is a very expensive program that offers halfway coverage to half of the people who need it."

Some opponents, coming from the other direction, claim the ACA amounts to "socialized medicine." Of all criticisms, this is the most mistaken. A program is socialist when the government employs its workers and owns the equipment. You may be surprised to learn we've long operated socialist programs. Police and fire departments function exactly this way, as does military medicine and the Veterans Administration. Under the ACA, the government employs no practitioners. They remain independent contractors, exactly the same arrangement as under private insurance.

Another common objection, that the ACA will "ration" healthcare, is valid. As a matter of fact, no system can survive without "rationing." If insurance didn't exist at all and we had to pay cash for every service, we'd compare what we want with what we could afford: we'd "ration" our care ourselves. That is, we'd set boundaries, judging whether the care in question is worth the expense. Any third-party payer, whether private or government, must do the same. If it agreed to pay every claim, from eyelid lifts to Tarot readings, it would go belly-up in its first month. A viable plan necessarily ranks healthcare interventions on a continuum from "basic" to "inessential," and then decides where to draw the lines. Certainly physicians and patients should participate in that discussion, asking what defines legitimate coverage . . .

. . . and what amounts to "waste." Currently, for example, 30 percent of Medicare's expenditures cover care in patients' final year. Much of that goes toward unbelievably expensive but predictably futile attempts to postpone death. If doctors were to conduct thorough end-of-life conversations with these families before the final crisis, much wasteful expense, not to mention suffering, could be avoided.

In an ideal system, a patient would obtain necessary care without interference from any third party, and with only minimal paperwork. The Taiwanese government, for example, covers 99 percent of its population with a program funded by general taxes, premiums based on the payroll tax, and some out-of-pocket payments. Most doctors operate as private contractors. Taiwanese simply flash their computerized wallet card and get treated. In 2010 their life expectancy was the same as that of Americans, and their healthcare costs were one-third less.

In comparison, the ACA allows much of our current crippling complexity. It lets the system remain festooned with hundreds of private insurance companies, thousands of incompatible forms, and an impenetrable jungle of policies and regulations. The navigational challenges and paperwork demands impact doctors and patients alike, diluting rather than strengthening their relationship. Doctors continue to spend scandalous stretches of time (experts estimate 20 percent of their work week) simply trying to obtain remuneration for services already performed. And patients, for their part, spend long periods either trying to understand insurance verbiage or listening to recorded music while holding for "service" representatives.

There's little evidence the ACA will limit the demand for new, ever more expensive technologies. As they proliferate, doctors and patients will use them, so costs will rise, along with premiums, deductibles, and copays. This isn't the fault of the ACA; it would occur with any plan, given our current thinking about healthcare. The only way we'll defuse accelerating expense is by heeding the advice of experts like John Knowles, M.D. (1926–1979), late President of the Rockefeller Foundation and Medical Director of Massachusetts General Hospital:

> The people have been led to believe that national health insurance, more doctors, and greater use of high-cost hospital-based technologies will improve their health. Unfortunately, none of them will. The next major advances in the health of the American people will come from the assumption of individual responsibility for one's own health and a necessary change in the life style of a majority of Americans.

That will take time, of course, and national effort. Meanwhile I find comfort in Winston Churchill's observation: "Leave it to the Americans to do the right thing . . . after they've tried all the wrong ones."

CHAPTER 18

Help Is On the Way

Our healthcare system was once the world's finest. We want to believe it still is, but it's getting harder to ignore its decline. During biomedicine's successful century, qualms about its emphasis on objectivity remained discreetly quiet until studies began to disclose its diminishing, however increasingly expensive, returns. Critics who looked beyond its cost especially declaimed its impersonality, noting that the patient and doctor, healthcare's vital center, had shrunk into vapid "consumers" and "providers." In reviewing Dr. Victoria Sweet's book *God's Hotel*, physician-author Danielle Ofri wrote, "I can't tell you exactly when it happened, but sometime in the past two decades, the practice of medicine was insidiously morphed into the delivery of health care."

Resistance to healthcare's decay has been mounting. One response is "Slow Medicine," deliberate deceleration as counterpoint to biomedicine's obsessive haste. A culture's healthcare style necessarily reflects its values, and to put it briefly, we're a society of sprinters. How we love speed. We want what we want, now. Fast food and instant coffee. Real-time communication. One-night stands. Multitasking. Zero to sixty in five seconds. Jet travel. Immediate cures. Rapidity is justified sometimes, as when addressing bacterial meningitis or hemorrhage. But as healthcare's default tempo, fast-forward leaves much unaddressed.

Patients with chronic conditions and at the end of life, for example, find substantial benefit in clinicians who take a breath, step back to admit a wider perspective, think about the whole situation, and discuss issues fully. In other words, practitioners who, rather than "deliver healthcare," practice caring medicine.

Other reform approaches accentuate meaning, intimacy, compassion, or the well-being of practitioners and caregivers. The Right Care Alliance[1] a project of the Lown Institute, emphasizes attentive restraint: "We seek to do as much as possible *for* the patient and as little as possible *to* the patient."

Henry Thoreau observed, "There are as many paths to the center as there are radii in a circle." These various approaches to healthcare reform are mutually congruent and now penetrating one another, steadily integrating into a practical transformation that's spreading through much of the United States.

I'll describe several such projects, purposely limiting my list to examples within a few hours' drive of my home in Northern California. If they interest you, it won't be hard to find your own local counterparts.

Each of these programs' creators was motivated by a single, identifiable personal event: a comment, a touch, a situation that reignited some indelible truth. (In the first chapter, you may recall, I mentioned my childhood experience of feeling healed when my doctor simply touched me.) They launched their innovations from their hearts, not from industrial focus groups or a business plan.

Finding Meaning in Medicine

Rachel Naomi Remen was trained as a pediatrician, and arguably more thoroughly as a patient. In her teens she developed Crohn's Disease, an inflammatory gastrointestinal disorder, and over time endured nine operations.

Sensing that some hospital staff behaved as though she were abnormal, defective, or even unclean, she sank into depression. Then one nurse acted differently. She related to Dr. Remen not as a patient, but as just another person, laughing with her and physically touching her. Now, decades later, this nurse is likely unaware that she helped her patient realize that sick or not, she was whole and strong.

As she practiced medicine, Dr. Remen recognized that whole and strong wasn't the self-image professional training imparts to medical students. Their hypercompetitive environment persuades them that they can never know enough or do enough. When patients claim their doctor is arrogant, they may actually be witnessing the doctor's defense against feeling perennially inadequate.

It's as though we've forgotten the ancient advice, "Physician, heal thyself." In order to heal her colleagues—and patients as well—Dr. Remen founded the Institute for the Study of Health & Illness (ISHI) in 1991 in Bolinas, California.[1] You can find samples of the wisdom informing her work in her two best-selling books, *Kitchen Table Wisdom* (1996) and *My Grandfather's Blessings* (2001).

One program Dr. Remen developed at ISHI is The Healer's Art, a course offered to first- and second-year medical students at more than eighty American medical schools and seven schools in other countries. It offers ". . . a safe learning environment for a personal in-depth exploration of the time-honored values of service, healing relationship, reverence for life, and compassionate care."

Another ISHI program, Finding Meaning in Medicine, helps practicing physicians achieve greater satisfaction by finding the deeper meaning always inherent in their work.

One FMM group (there are many that meet periodically around the country) invited me to participate in a session. The meeting began, unlike other medical gatherings, with a short meditation and the reading of a poem. This ritual marked the ensuing two hours as extraordinary, a withdrawal from the daily world into a special dimension characterized by slowness, thoughtfulness, depth, and respect.

Participants are invited to tell a story from their experience of training and practice related to the topic of the evening—in this case it was "light"—and are encouraged to listen "generously," accept-ingly, without judgment or criticism. This ambiance conjures a degree of vulnerability unusual among physician groups.

FMM's lifeblood, understandably, is trust, so strict confidentiality reigns. The meeting's host asked me not to speak or write about anything that transpired, nor to contact any participant afterward for further discussion. It feels advisable, however, to describe the conduct of the meeting in a general way, as doctors who have never heard of FMM can at least learn such gatherings are possible.

Some docs told stories of profound fulfillment in their practice. Others related tales of tragedy and painful dissatisfaction. This was extraordinary, as medical conversations in hospital settings con-sist mainly of terminology and numbers, all else being deemed extraneous. It felt as though those long cautioned to be silent about their inner worlds had permission to speak here and hear one another, and to reaffirm that they're not alone in their struggles, their dreams, and their purpose.

For me, the meeting was a revelation. When given permission to speak subjectively, physicians can be consummate artists. Hearing them, I joyfully remembered what exemplary beings many of us docs are, committed to service and medicine's magic, and how sad it is when we, along with patients, are injured by industrial practice.

SCHWARTZ CENTER ROUNDS

If doctors can speak their hearts in secure sessions like Finding Meaning in Medicine, can they speak as openly within their more public hospitals? That's what Schwartz Center Rounds aims for.

Ken Schwartz was a lawyer who contracted lung cancer at the age of forty. He exercised and ate healthily, and never smoked. While under treatment, he found that his favorite caregivers were those who were fully present to patients. As he put it, they made "the unbearable bearable." Just before he died in 1995, he founded The Schwartz Center for Compassionate Healthcare.

The Center operates a number of projects intended to make the unbearable bearable. One is Schwartz Center Rounds, a world different from standard hospital meetings in that this isn't about patients, but those who contact patients. These Rounds focus on *their feelings*, the unbearable that practitioners nonetheless try to bear.

Physicians—and others who labor amid suffering—commonly repress the emotions that arise in their work. Schwartz Rounds offers them permission to emote. And here it's more challenging than Finding Meaning in Medicine, since it occurs not in a secure private living room, but in as safe and supportive a venue as can be arranged in a hospital.

After I'd seen a few Schwartz Center videos, I started boosting the idea in our little local hospital. Other souls got interested, and soon we were signed up. In 2013 we held our first Rounds.

Our opening presentation concerned Gordon, a doctor on our hospital staff who'd died three months earlier from congestive heart failure. For the first ten minutes of this session, a nurse and doctor who'd cared for him described his medical course and their involvement in it.

Randy, the nurse, said, "He was obviously failing. His meds lost efficacy. He was swelling up more, and had trouble breathing. We told him treatment wasn't going well, and asked what he thought we ought to do. I figured that as a doctor himself, he knew how grave the situation was. I hoped he'd just ask for morphine and other palliation, but no. He wanted everything done. He told me more than once, 'You think I'm dying, but I'll show you. I've gotta get home, back to work. I have things to do.'"

Randy continued, "I wanted to say, 'Gordon, look: you know how serious this is. We can't do much to treat your heart anymore. It looks like our best efforts will only make you suffer more.'

But you don't say that to patients. That's the conversation we ought to have before they get so sick. So I was really frustrated."

Gordon's doctor, Alice, said, "I found myself getting angry at him. His care choices were making things worse for everyone. The nurses were slaving around the clock for him, which stole time from less sick patients.

"When Gordon's heart finally stopped, we had to follow his instructions. We called a 'Code Blue.' The crash team came. I intubated him and began giving him CPR. When I looked up, I saw all these eyes, the people I work with, looking at me so sadly. Everyone knew this was a charade. If I'd been alone, I'd have slowed down or even pronounced him. I hate when I'm caught in a situation like that. In a way, I feel like I didn't do much of a service for Gordon, or actually, he didn't let me. I want to tell him, 'You made me disappointed in myself, Gordon. I'm ashamed of being so manipulated. To tell you the truth, I feel abused.' No, that sounds kind of cruel. It's not Gordon . . ."

As facilitator, I thanked Randy and Alice, commended them on their honesty, and asked our audience, "How did their stories make you feel?"

The floodgates opened. Doctor after nurse after technician said how sad or angry they felt—not only about what they'd just heard, but other stories they'd lived. They told tales of aggravation, sadness, resentment. A few choked up or cried. Some commented that they'd never spoken of these incidents and feelings before, having assumed early in their careers that professionalism required emotional reserve. The evaluations submitted afterward were replete with comments like, "I didn't know doctors had such a hard time with these issues," "I need to listen more deeply," and, "I feel like I can speak more freely to colleagues."

In Schwartz Rounds since then, I've noticed a fascinating phenomenon. When doctors first visit, most look a bit confused, as though they're thinking, "What's going on here? This isn't like any medical rounds I've been to. Where's the PowerPoint? Why is Susie crying?"

To the medical mind, Schwartz Rounds is initially foreign territory, but docs who keep attending eventually go native. On their second visit, its very strangeness causes their scientific drive to kick in. If I read their thoughts accurately, they're saying to themselves, "These people are my respected biomedical cohort, not the civilians I'd expect all this emotion from, so who's odd here, them or me?" They'll think about this question and likely speak their own truth in the next Rounds.

The Schwartz Center has evolved a remarkably effective Rounds template. It suggests, for example, that all hospital staff with any patient contact—including office, dietary, maintenance, and security—be invited, not just medical professionals. The Center insists that food be served, as dining together promotes community. Attendees are encouraged to pass on stories for their educational riches, but must disguise details and identities. Problem-solving, which is standard strategy in medical rounds, is banned from Schwartz Rounds: here we aren't problems to be solved, but humans making our wayward way. Some participants express gratitude that the Center discourages resolving issues raised in Rounds, and instead expects discussion to continue throughout the hospital afterward, indefinitely.

"DOCTORING" COURSE

Four-year-old Eddie S drowned in his backyard swimming pool. EMTs managed to reactivate his heart, but emergency department physicians determined he was brain-dead. Now his parents are waiting in the corridor. They haven't been told anything.

Mr. S paces the floor, flexing his fists. He growls to his wife, "Now look what you've done. You had to be on the phone, right? You couldn't look out into the backyard even once!"

Bent forward in a plastic chair, Ms. S holds her face in her hands, crying.

Dr. N introduces himself and, as he ushers the parents into a small conference room, regards them carefully.

He regards them as he would in real life . . . which this isn't.

Dr. N is a junior medical student in his early twenties, and the Ss are actors playing roles in the "Doctoring" course at the University of California at Davis School of Medicine.

This is Dr. N's third year in the course, so he has tools. He noted that Mr. S's scowl appears to be his daily face, and that Ms. S seems oddly accustomed to weeping. So there are two problems here: little Eddie's death is the awful frosting on a long-term misery cake.

Taking a seat, he pauses, breathes, and says, "Would you like to sit down, Mr. S?"

Twitching with anger, Dad takes a chair.

Dr. N says, "Would you like a little more time alone? I can come back."

"No," Mom says without looking up. "Tell us."

"I'm afraid I have bad news. Eddie made it to the hospital and he's on life support now. But his brain went without oxygen too long. He's brain-dead."

Dad says, "But he's going to come around okay, isn't he?"

A long pause. "No, he isn't. 'Brain-dead' and 'life support' means we're keeping him alive artificially. That's the best we can do. And we can't do it indefinitely."

Mom screams in pain. "Oh, God, Eddie's dead!"

"He is not!" he screams at his wife. "Come on, doc. I know what you guys can do, restart hearts and all that. You bring him back."

"I'm sorry, Mr. S. Is there someone we can call? Would you like to talk with another doctor or a counselor?"

There can be no happy ending here. Even though it's fictitious, the scene leaves everyone shaken. Relating dreadful news to relatives is an inevitable part of medical practice. It can be done brusquely or with kindness.

My own training in such delicate communication was exactly zero. Had I, as a junior student, been appointed to break the news about a real-life Eddie, I might not have even thought to bring the Ss to a private room. I might not have sat down with them. I might not even have looked carefully enough to see them. I probably would have told them, "I'm sorry. He didn't survive," and then left the room.

The doctoring sessions feature two faculty members, eight to ten junior students, and a senior student. The senior at the Eddie session was a surgeon-to-be. Surgeons aren't known as warm and fuzzy players in the trade, yet this one asked her colleagues, more than once, "How does that make you feel?"

Another session began with an instructor saying, "As you know, your first two med school years were about facts. It's logical and memorizable. Now, in your third year, you get the hard part, human beings. They're quirky and irrational. They're unpredictable. Sometimes, in practice, they'll spray you with their fear or anger or sometimes even with praise. You'll believe it's about you, and it hardly ever is. They live in their own worlds, which you'll never enter, so can be mysterious. The art of medicine, then, consists of connecting in the fog."

In this session, students witnessed one of their fellows, again an actor, steal a prescription pad from an instructor's desk. She clearly had a drug problem. The student assigned to deal with the issue immediately grasped that her task required a difficult mixture of tact, firmness, and compassion.

She said to the actor, "I saw you take that prescription pad."

"Oh, no big deal. I needed to get uppers for my diagnosis practical. Everybody does it."

"Don't you recognize that's dishonest?"

The actor raised the ante. "Look, it's a common practice. You can't turn me in for that. You'll wreck my career before it even starts."

The student gulped. Her body language said, "There but for the grace of God . . ." But she quickly regained her footing. "You need counseling. That's what the school offers. I'm sorry if that affects your career, but taking that pad was your doing, not mine."

Addressing the actor's every objection and rationalization, the student eventually got her to agree to see the school's counselor.

Since the 1970s I attended I-don't-know-how-many classes and workshops that were rudimentary predecessors of the doctoring course. I learned what might be called "bedside manner technique:" how to make eye contact, where to sit, when not to speak. These courses mainly helped me get clearer about what I sought, which wasn't any technique, but a style. I longed for a way of being that came naturally and felt easy. In the final analysis, it's easier to be compassionate than to act compassionate. So are doctoring students simply learning technique or actually becoming more compassionate? Or does it matter?

I put that question to one of Doctoring's senior faculty, psychiatrist Dr. Nathan Fairman. He wears absent-minded apparel, an enviable thinker's brow, and a serious demeanor from which emerges plenty of straight-faced humor.

Nathan told me, "Some students will only be able to fake it till they make it. Some other students are genuinely and openly compassionate, but they learn not to let this intimate quality 'interfere' with patient care. The students who need to fake it get a chance in Doctoring to get better at faking it, while the naturally compassionate students learn to give themselves permission to be authentic."

Nathan started out as a bird biologist, living months at a time on the austere Farallon Islands, off the San Francisco coast.

With his wife-to-be in graduate school then, the notion of continuing his own education enticed him. His father was a physician, and though he says he held no great yearning for the medical profession, he nevertheless enrolled in pre-med courses and finally U.C. Davis' medical school.

He took the Doctoring course as a student, but its ideals sometimes conflicted with what he saw in actual practice. Despite widespread lip service to "compassion" and "caring for the whole patient," visits were limited to twelve minutes, and a glance around the clinic waiting room revealed piles of pharmaceutical industry literature and, Nathan recalls with a chuckle, a wall clock designed around a garish Viagra logo. By his third year, he was seriously disillusioned.

As a resident he was further chagrined by his peers' reactions to a birth within their group. They surrounded the new father and congratulated him, partly for the happy event and more, it seemed to Nathan, for choosing to come to work the day of the birth. What a dedicated doc! What a teammate and professional! Amid the back-slapping, Nathan thought, "No. Wrong."

He stayed on, crediting three faculty mentors for inspiring him to believe the system might be redeemable. He completed his psychiatry residency, earned a master's degree in public health, and got certified in palliative medicine. Nathan is patient, aware that the change he seeks in healthcare's character is slow but sure.

Other schools are inventing their own "doctoring" or "nursing" courses, by the way. In Massachusetts, Martha Keochareon,[2] a fifty-nine-year-old woman who'd graduated from Holyoke Community College nursing school in 1993, was dying from pancreatic cancer. She asked her alma mater if they'd be interested in having their students see her to more closely explore the dying process. They were indeed interested, and Ms. Keochareon was delighted to teach the students they sent.

One instructor observed that when students ran out of medical questions, they practiced what she called ". . . therapeutic communication, the way we've learned in school and haven't applied enough. They say, 'I'm glad to be with you; you must be frustrated; you look uncomfortable.' And they let the patient just talk and talk and talk . . ."

TELEPHONE CAREGIVER SUPPORT GROUP

Having collaborated with Marlene M. von Friederichs-Fitzwater, PhD, MPH, on health communication projects over the last twenty-five years, I'm continually astonished at her commitment, patience, and her unceasing flow of innovative ideas.

In the late 1970s, Marlene, then a single mother of four sons, was diagnosed with cancer. Unable to take time off work, she squeezed in treatment as she could. She felt most professionals she consulted diminished or dismissed her, especially as her prognosis worsened. One doctor responded to her questions by saying, "Honey, leave all that to me."

Only her family physician stayed closely connected. One day he visited her hospital room, sat on her bed, and said, "This is shit, isn't it?" She realized then, with this contrasting example, that something was "horribly wrong" with the medical system. She took a vow at that moment: "If I survive, I want to give back. No one with cancer should have this isolating experience."

After regaining her health, she returned to school, earned a PhD, and founded the non-profit Health Communication Research Institute in Sacramento. She also taught doctor-patient communication to first-year medical students and developed and taught communication classes to pre-med and nursing students at another local university. Passionately concerned with patients' experiences, she is just as involved with their caregivers, whom she also considers patients.

Two years ago, she began to wonder about cancer caregivers who lived too rurally or were too busy to attend a support group meeting. So she started a monthly phone-in group. Soon doctors, traditionally unequipped to treat caregivers, began referring them to Marlene.

I participated in several of Marlene's phone conferences with caregivers. As in in-person groups, people's initial responses are often revelational: "I thought I was the only one going through this!" When I told Marlene I prefer in-person groups, where body language is visible and physical touch possible, she replied, "Sure, but some people feel more comfortable with anonymity. They're free to be more honest with like minds who don't actually know them."

Marlene lists some of her caregiver program's accomplishments: "They learn what questions to ask and where to find resources. They learn practical assertiveness. They recognize that they're patients, too, deserving of respect and treatment. They learn the all-important principle of creating personal boundaries and taking care of themselves. They create realistic expectations."

In one of these phone sessions, Barbara, a resident of remote Alpine County (population 1,200) called the toll-free number to join Marlene and a half-dozen other phoned-in caregivers.

She told the group, "My husband has stage four cancer and is now under hospice care. His brother and sister-in-law live an hour away and insist on seeing him regularly, usually along with their kids. They're sponges, these people. They move into our home, make meals for themselves—and only for themselves—and never do a lick of work. I thought I was a caregiver for just my husband; now I find I'm doing it for his whole family."

Marlene said, "Gee, that sounds really tough. How do you feel about it, Barbara?"

"Well, I try to be a good wife and hostess. I cook and clean and do the medications and shopping and . . ."

"Barbara, how do you feel about it?"

"It's a lot of work. I know my husband appreciates it, but none of these other . . ."

"Barbara, how do you feel about it?"

"Oh. Well, kind of upset, I guess."

Karen, calling from Sierra County (population 3,240) asked, "Upset? What does that mean?"

"Well, I guess kind of put out."

Marlene asks, "Barbara, is it hard for you to say you're angry?"

"Oh, Marlene, I've never been able to do that."

"You want to try? Just say it. Say, 'I'm angry.' See how it feels."

"Uh. I'm . . . uh . . . I'm angry."

"Can you say it and sound angry?"

"I'm angry. Angry! Angry angry angry! Who the hell do those people think they are?"

"Barbara," Marlene said, "please keep us posted."

This sounds like Schwartz Center Rounds, doesn't it? Here, though, the participants aren't professional caregivers, but patients, actually family members suffering the same subtle burden we place on all caregivers—the imperative to be dedicated beyond even voicing one's own suffering. Treatment is no different from what we use with patients: tell me how it is for you. I won't try to fix you, only accompany you to the heart of your pain.

SPIRITUAL CARE

Until a few years ago, the hospital chaplains I met were a glum Dickensian bunch. They may as well have worn black stovepipe hats and carried a shovel along with their bible. Recently, though, a new generation has taken over.

More positive and intimate, their *modus operandi* clearly favors listening over speaking. Our local hospital's chaplain, David Swetman, is of this breed. Constantly paying close but relaxed attention, he's obviously more interested in whomever he's with than in any message he'd consider delivering. His twinkling eye and mischievous sense of humor express an engaging blend of reverence and irreverence.

David grew up in a fundamentalist Christian family. In the mid-1970s he helped found a church in the Chicago suburbs that today boasts fifteen thousand weekly attendees. As the church grew and requests for counseling increased, he thought it would be useful to obtain official credentials, so he earned a master's degree in counseling at Northwestern University.

When instructors told him he had to clarify clients' issues, he realized he needed to view people through a wider-angle lens. He gradually moved out of the church and into private practice, then into a variety of interests, including film production and Wall Street finance. When he was forty-two, his Wall Street partner died in a freak accident, leading David to ponder what he was doing with his own finite life.

Moving to Sacramento, he volunteered at Sutter Health Hospice. When they needed a new chaplain, David expressed interest, explaining that in addition to being a psychotherapist, he'd helped found a church. Sutter put him through a one-year training program, after which our community's hospital hired him.

David is unusual among chaplaincy department managers in maintaining a corps of volunteer assistants, known unofficially around the hospital as the "Balm Squad." He recruits six to eight at a time and prepares them, in thirteen weekly two-hour sessions, to provide what he calls "spiritual care."

David doesn't behave accidentally, and I think I know why he chose that phrase. Twenty years ago I participated in a daylong workshop conducted by our local hospice. In one exercise, we separated into groups of eight to answer and discuss a questionnaire about our own beliefs. One item read, "Agree or Disagree: My religion is important to me." I crossed out "religion" and wrote in "spirituality." In the ensuing discussion, it turned out all eight of us had done exactly that. Perhaps broad-spectrum spirituality—openness to a wide variety of views—is a growing "religion."

The flyer David distributes to patients and families includes this statement:

> You think. You feel. You communicate. You have relationships. You have a style, a sense of humor, an attitude and an approach to life. Perhaps you have deep religious beliefs or a strong connection to God; perhaps you have none. It is all these non-physical parts of you that make up your spiritual self.

And significantly, it is in exactly these non-physical parts that suffering resides, and where it can be treated.

David currently deploys twenty-five of his graduates throughout the hospital. They've undergone hospital orientations, TB testing, several immunizations, background checks, and even fingerprinting. Wearing maroon "Spiritual Care Volunteer" vests, they spend four-hour weekly shifts responding to patients and families who request meetings.

One volunteer told me about seeing a woman who was about to undergo elective surgery. "She asked to see me because she was nervous," he said. "That was obvious: she was tight, even shaking a little. I asked her what I could do to help. She said, 'Would you just lay your hand on my forehead?' Of course, I did. In three minutes she was asleep."

David and his recent trainees permitted me to attend one of their training sessions. He began, "What is suffering?"

The trainees offered their opinions.

"It's pain, but more like emotional pain. Is emotional pain real, by the way?"

"Suffering's just feeling awful. Some is worse than others."

"Suffering is the decoration we put on pain."

"What do you mean?"

"Well, you get a headache. But you've had cancer, so what's your first thought about the headache? 'Oh oh. Cancer's back.' And you go downhill from there. 'I'm circling the drain,' you think. 'Better get that power of attorney done. Should I buy a plot? Go to church?' You've got nine toes in the ground, and all from this symptom, which most likely is just a plain old headache. That's why you see that bumper sticker, 'Pain is inevitable; suffering is optional.'"

David asks, "Well, isn't that a normal reaction? And what if the headache really is a cancer recurrence?"

As the conversation evolves over months, trainees absorb the notion that sickness involves suffering, which is individually unique and treatable. In other sessions, the group discusses perceptions versus beliefs, attitudes inherited from their birth families, and other predispositions that might inadvertently color their interaction with patients and families. Eventually they get to the issues popularly associated with chaplaincy, such as theology and prayer.

David says, "I call this training 'Healing My Relationship With Myself.' When you counsel someone, the counseling isn't about you. You're only the tool, the vehicle. So you need to enter that room cleanly, aware of issues that might push your buttons. You can't have any agenda. Even if all you do is listen and hold space with minimal speaking, that's often enough."

If I'd learned to "Heal My Relationship With Myself' in medical school, I'd have saved thousands spent later on therapy. In fact, the only people for whom such training wouldn't be useful are those who won't experience suffering in themselves or others.

CHAPTER 19

The Coming Change

decade ago I visited a revered grandfather of the compassion-in-healthcare movement. During an afternoon with him in his light-filled library, a former Brooklyn brewery, I asked him whether he expected American healthcare to become tangibly more humane during his lifetime.

He laughed. "Absolutely not. I'm pretty old, so it'd have to happen next week. By the way, how old are you?"

I told him. He looked me up and down and said, "Not in your lifetime, either."

As of this writing we're both still kicking, so don't hold your breath for the coming compassion *tsunami*. Yet its arrival is certain.

The dismal news is that biomedicine's dispassionate, high-tech style is clearly unsustainable. The good news is that innovative programs promoting more personal healthcare are in vibrant bloom. These programs aren't healthcare industry products; they come from patients, doctors, and caregivers.

Evolution will occur not from the top down, as from legal dictate or financial incentive, but via our own daily behavior. Most docs are too inhibited by their profession's implicit rules to change healthcare, so the mission will fall mainly to patients, individually and in movements. To paraphrase Arlo Guthrie's "Alice's Restaurant," just one person acting imaginatively may be psychotic; two doing it are a *folie à deux*, three are a conspiracy, but four comprise a subculture. Here are a few steps you, as a patient, can take.

Frame your relationship with doctors realistically

We docs are well trained and competent in certain areas. But we're neither omniscient nor omnipotent. And patients, however passive or ignorant they envision themselves, are in fact the only authorities on their own sensations, beliefs, and behavior.

Given the mutual respect these expertises deserve, you'll enhance your care by crafting a horizontal relationship with physicians. Pediatrician Robert Mendelsohn offered an apt prophecy in his 1979 book, *Confessions of a Medical Heretic*: "We physicians will come down off our pedestals as soon as patients get up off their knees."

If you believe, as I do, that our current system mistreats caregivers as well as patients, you'll see your doc through more compassionate eyes. He or she may be figuratively and even literally dying to enjoy more personal relationships with patients, yet hamstrung by training and the demands of overseers to initiate it.

So it's up to you. Glance around the medical office. Note the massive paperwork, the insurance hassles, the rush, the inevitable missing information—collectively the frustrations of industrial medicine—and return your attention to the only other proper occupant of the examining room, your physician. Imagine the bond with your doctor as a kind of friendship. So ask: How are you doing, Doc? Let me tell you about my life, and by the way, how's yours going? Most doctors yearn for this closeness. One of my medical classmates meets every new patient not by saying, "What's wrong?" but, "Tell me about yourself." Another doctor told me how he's chosen doctors for himself. "The three A's," he said. "Amiability, accessibility, and ability. *In that order.*"

Practice informed consent

A medical principle venerable enough for Latin is *primum non nocere*, above all do no harm. Ideally, we docs want to avoid collateral damage. At the same time, though, we're aware that our treatments can indeed cause harm. In fact, no drug or procedure can be said to be entirely risk-less, which is why we also value a sister principle, *informed consent*. Given that a drug, say, can be helpful or hazardous or both, doctors need to fully inform patients, and for their part, patients need to make decisions from full education.

That's not always possible, since even in the best of circumstances, information is limited. For some surgical procedures and newer drugs, there may not be much known yet, especially about long-term effects. Sometimes, from desperation, you just don't want to know, and would rather take a leap of faith, such as deliberately not reading the entire scary statement you're required to sign when you're admitted to a hospital.

Before taking any medical step, learn about it. Talk with patients who've decided for and against what you're contemplating. Never hesitate to get a second medical opinion.

Above all, avoid medical advertising. Mixtures of information, misinformation, distraction, and omission, drug ads directed at patients are illegal in every country except New Zealand and the United States. Remember, they're not created by health-zealous copywriters, but marketers who naturally put their best foot forward while concealing their worst. They aim to attract customers with graphics of ecstatic patients reveling in the success of some product, or with a compelling celebrity as salesperson.

Pfizer pharmaceuticals, for example, spent $258 million on an advertising campaign for the cholesterol-lowering drug Lipitor featuring Dr. Robert Jarvik, inventor the Jarvik-7 artificial heart. His endorsement looked authoritative until critics pointed out that he was neither a cardiologist nor licensed anywhere to practice medicine. Pfizer soon withdrew the ads.

Keep in mind that no drugs are without side effects. If that magazine photo of the woman joyously cartwheeling after whomping her arthritis with Jointbliss™ attracts you, turn the page to read the list of the drug's potential hazards. It's lengthy, as the manufacturer is required to publish every known side effect and toxicity. You might temper your disenchantment by thinking, "Respiratory arrest? That must not be very common." But each effect actually impacted someone, and the longer the list, the more likely one will affect you.

An even better reason to ignore these ads is that they reinforce the popular yet erroneous notion that drugs or surgery or some clinic or doctor or alternative practitioner can fix whatever's wrong with you. It'd be helpful if they were balanced by other ads recommending, say, review of your lifestyle. Indeed, "public service announcements" in the media advise Don't Smoke, Drink Moderately, Take a Walk, and Wear Your Seatbelt, but as they're produced by under-funded organizations, they're feeble in comparison to slick corporate copy.

Informed consent means considering what you've responsibly gathered from all sources. Depending on the situation, almost any drug or procedure might be suitable. Choose it only after weighing potential consequences.

Be skeptical about medical technology

Regarding new drugs and procedures, doctors advise one another, "Don't be the first or last to adopt it." American pharmaceutical history, for example, is rich in recalls. In the 1940s, the synthetic hormone diethylstilbestrol (DES) prevented thousands of pregnant women at risk from miscarrying. It worked like a dream, but proved nightmarish two or more decades later, when many of these women's young adult children developed genital cancers.

Another drug, Thalidomide, was prescribed in Europe as a sedative and to alleviate morning sickness in pregnant women. In the United States, manufacturer Richardson-Merrell pressured the Food and Drug Administration to approve it, but a single

FDA pharmacologist, Dr. Frances Kelsey, blocked the way, reso-
lutely insisting further studies were needed. The drug was never
approved in this country.[1] Months after Thalidomide became an
over-the-counter drug in Germany in 1957, thousands of babies
were born with phocomelia, severe congenital foreshortening of
their limbs.

Consider the mind as real as the body

You know by now I enjoy posing impertinent questions. When I
ask folks, "Where is your mind located?" they usually point to their
head. That's a reasonable choice considering the head's concentra-
tion of sense organs. Yet if we recognize the existence of "body
language," we know part of the mind resides below the neck and
continually expresses itself without cerebral consultation.

Some of that expression consists of the glandular and muscular
dysfunctions that steer toward overt illness. That can be a difficult
principle to accept, since it invokes the specter of our complicity
in getting sick. The question, "Did I create my illness?" can raise
a bucket of guilt, brimming with issues we'd rather not confront.
For that reason, plenty of intelligent people prefer to deny the
mind's role in illness.

My friend Dale learned from his doctor that his troubling
fatigue resulted from a cardiac arrhythmia. Instead of beating
with effective steadiness, his heart threw in an occasional prema-
ture, wobbly contraction that diminished blood circulation. He
was given a drug that partly corrected it. When I asked him how
his life was going, he mentioned a couple of areas of intense recent
stress, but insisted, "My heart thing isn't about stress. You can see
it on my EKG. This is *real*."

Excuse me, but it's all real. Biomedicine's greatest error, I
think, is defining imagination as imaginary. The body is real, the
mind is real, and their mutual influence is real.

Don't assume illness is a random affliction

We generally believe sickness comes from haphazard chance. But whether *anything* is random is questionable. At the end of his life, Albert Einstein concluded that pattern is universal, that God "doesn't roll dice." Maybe he was right, maybe not, but considering that the entire history of science amounts to teasing order from apparent chaos, our penchant for perceiving illness as random is surprising.

I say, "I caught a cold," as though the cold had been a predator drone that mindlessly picked me out of the crowd. The image begs the koan, "What did my cold look like before I caught it?"

To see illness as random affliction is only one view among alternatives. Seeing it as a verb, for example—I'm colding—raises questions that randomness can't. Why am I colding now? Why in this way? Did some event injure my immunity? Was I exposed to toxins? Does this illness remove me from a destructive setting or get me the attention I craved? If I thought my colding might be a form of body language, what would it be saying? Simply having a doctor exorcise the intruder may prove successful, but at the cost of learning something about myself. Choosing to see meaning in my illness doesn't exclude taking the medical route in addition. It's possible to reap existential healing along with cure. (I rush to mention that sometimes being sick is all we can do, and seeking its personal significance at that time is an intrusive burden.)

Get more comfortable with dying

There's no getting around the subject. Novelist William Saroyan is said to have remarked on his deathbed, "I know everyone's going to die, but I thought in my case they might make an exception." As it turned out, they didn't.

That ominous advice, "Get your affairs in order," assumes, often correctly, that we've postponed the chore in a wishful bid for immortality. If we don't think about it, it won't happen.

Regarding death as too morbid or too messy to talk about will eventually cause us, and our loved ones, trouble. I've seen any number of family donnybrooks around deathbeds, as relatives wrestle with weighty decisions via their own long-held feelings instead of the wishes of the dying. "You just say that because you're itching for your inheritance." "You're acting crazy, as usual." "You never loved Dad anyway." Obviously, such arguments only fore-stall decisions and besides, don't help Dad a bit. So as difficult as it might feel at first, find a way to discuss your preferences around your eventual departure with those around you.

Freeing yourself from dread of the *D* word will likely change you. Elisabeth Kübler-Ross, author of the classic *On Death and Dying*, pointed out that once we deal with our fear of death, we live our life instead of grimly clinging to it. What would you want done or not done if you become too sick to state your wishes? Who would you want to make healthcare decisions in your stead? What does "do everything possible" actually mean, and conversely, what degree of degradation and indignity are you prepared to tolerate?

Improve your health by improving your life

The next time you see one of those lists labeled "Ten Changes to Make if You Have Cancer," or "Ten Ways to Avoid Depression," or "Ten Things You Can Do to Prolong Your Life," notice that they're identical: Eat sensibly. Exercise. Nurture rewarding relationships. Find fulfilling work. Take time to relax. Whatever else these tips accomplish, they describe a good life in general and don't need to relate to illness or longevity at all.

Why wouldn't we want to live well now instead of waiting until we get sick and then using that as an excuse to upgrade? Alfred Adler, a psychiatric colleague of Sigmund Freud, is said to have asked his patients, "How would you behave if you were cured?" After they answered him, he'd say, "Then why don't you act that way now?"

Adler's question is silly and at the same time the most useful one we can ask ourselves, especially once we accept that we won't be here forever. That's why conversations in cancer support groups don't focus on the weather and commute times. The diagnosis bears the message, "Your days were always numbered; now that that's undeniable, how are you going to live out your remainder?"

What is "the good life," after all? As the sages say, if you can see the path it must not be yours. We must all go our unique way, and when undeniable mortality presses our face into the existential mirror, we make our most honest choices.

My French friend Marie developed chest pain. The emergency physician she saw confirmed that her coronary arteries were partly blocked, making her heart hurt.

"What's your diet like?" he asked.

"Oh, you know, paté, Camembert, that sort of thing."

He was horrified. "Don't you know that's all fat? For you, that's absolutely poison!"

"Maybe," she replied, "but I'm French. That's what I like, what I need, and who I am."

It's ten years later now, and Marie still enjoys her French diet and her life. Go figure.

Be proactive

Government won't help you address stress. A registered dietitian isn't going to drop by to remove the junk food from your pantry. You can't hire a television fitness star to exercise for you, or expect the AMA to render your doctor more personable. The mission is entirely yours, and frankly, that's the surest way toward healthcare progress.

Finally, consider healthcare reform primarily a moral rather than economic challenge

Industrial biomedicine's relative impotence in regard to chronic, lifestyle, and end-of-life disorders, along with its expense and impersonality, dissatisfies patients and doctors alike. Ask docs you know whether they think a seven-minute visit ending with the obligatory prescription is good medicine. Ask them whether a life-threatening operation rather than simple lifestyle change is good medicine. Ask them how they feel about faceless corporations and agencies controlling their practice. There's much wrong with the entire system—wrong meaning not just incorrect, but repugnant in its abuse of the principal parties.

Wrong though it is, we've all participated, so to some extent it expresses values we tolerate if not agree with. As we change course, individually and in appreciable numbers, so will our healthcare system. Stewart Brand, iconic innovator and founder of the *Whole Earth Catalog*, wrote, "You can't change a game by winning it or losing it. You can change it only by playing your own game, and if yours is better, people will play it." The new game isn't about money or technology or even science as much as the healing that results from intimacy. As the poet Rumi observed, "Through love, all pain is turned to medicine."

ACKNOWLEDGEMENTS

A book is something sculpted from nothing, so it's little wonder writers treasure a nurturing atmosphere. I'm grateful to author and visionary Peter Barnes,[1] founder of Mesa Refuge in Point Reyes, California, for my two-week residency. Lacking the silence and solitude of that writer's Eden, this book would still be vapor.

Meaningful reform of healthcare requires knowledge of its history. The most pertinent, even eye-opening narrative I've discovered is *Rockefeller Medicine Men* (University of California Press, 1979), authored by E. Richard Brown, late professor in UCLA's Fielding School of Public Health.

I'm grateful to the hundreds of people with whom I've worked in cancer support groups these thirty-plus years. They've offered insights into illness and treatment that are all but invisible within standard medical practice.

Fellow pilgrims on the path of restoring healthcare's humanity bestowed the encouragement, guidance, support, and participatory opportunities that helped me express initially hazy ideas. They include: Ruth Bolletino, PhD; Katy Butler; Eric Cassell, MD; Ladd Bauer, MD; Shannon Brownlee, MS; Nathan Fairman, MD, MPH; Marlene von Friederichs-Fitzwater, PhD, MPH; Pat Forman, MPH, MA; Phil Kerslake; Lawrence LeShan, PhD; Rachel Naomi Remen, MD; Chaplain David Swetman; and Matthew Zwerling, MD.

Thanks to Rob Wunderlich, who traversed otherwise impenetrable regions of cyberspace for me, and even gave me his office, and to Mark Wilson and Thomas Nigh for their acute editing skills.

My wife, Ronnie Paul, is my indispensable guide. Having come to equate healing with meticulous honesty (Ronnie is actually Veronica, Latin for "speaker of truth"), I pay her close attention since she not only says what's so, but always kindly, compassionately. She knows how to listen, too. As an interviewer, both amateur and professional, she draws astounding candor from others. What I've learned from her is the foundation of my work.

NOTES

Chapter 2

1. International Federation of Health Plans, "International Federation of Health Plans 2012 Comparative Price Report." https://static.squarespace.com/static/518a3cfee4b0a77d03a62c98/t/51dfd9f9e4b0d1d8067dcde2/1373624825901/2012

Chapter 3

1. Interestingly, Abraham Flexner eventually came around to Osler's view. In the 1920s he charged that ". . . Scientific medicine in America . . . is today sadly deficient in cultural and philosophic background." He wrote that ". . . the imposition of rigid standards by accrediting groups was making the medical curriculum a monstrosity," leaving medical students ". . . little time to stop, read, work, or think." In his later years, Flexner co-founded Princeton University's Institute for Advanced Study, recruiting as faculty the likes of Kurt Gödel, John von Neumann, and Albert Einstein.

Chapter 4

1. Laura Dolson, "Sugar's Many Disguises." About Health, September 16, 2014. http://lowcarbdiets.about.com/od/whattoeat/a/sugars.htm
2. Nicholas Confessore, "Minority Groups and Bottlers Team Up in Battles over Soda," *New York Times,* March 12, 2013. https://www.nytimes.com/2013/03/13/nyregion/behind-soda-industrys-win-a-phalanx-of-sponsored-minority-groups.html?pagewanted=all&_r=0

Chapter 5

1. Dean Ornish et al., "Can lifestyle changes reverse coronary heart disease? The Lifestyle Heart Trial." *Lancet* 1990 Jul 21;336(8708):129-33.

   http://www.ncbi.nlm.nih.gov/pubmed/1973470

2. American Psychiatric Association, "DSM-5 Development Task Force Members."

   http://www.dsm5.org/MeetUs/Pages/TaskForceMembers.aspx

3. Alan Schwarz, "Thousands of Toddlers Are Medicated for A.D.H.D., Report Finds, Raising Worries." *New York Times*, May 16, 2014.

   http://www.nytimes.com/2014/05/17/us/among-experts-scrutiny-of-attention-disorder-diagnoses-in-2-and-3-year-olds. html?ref=health&_r=4

4. Joel Lexchin, "The Role Of Sales Representatives In Driving Physicians' Off-Label Prescription Habits." Health Affairs Blog, June 19th, 2014.

   http://healthaffairs.org/blog/2014/06/19/ the-role-of-sales-representatives-in-driving-physi- cians-off-label-prescription-habits/?utm_source=rss&utm_ medium=rss&utm_campaign=the-role-of-sales-representa- tives-in-driving-physicians-off-label-prescription-habits

5. Henry Waxman, "The Lessons of Vioxx — Drug Safety and Sales." *New England Journal of Medicine* 352;25, June 23, 2005.

   http://www.nejm.org/doi/pdf/10.1056/NEJMp058136

6. Margaret Cronin Fisk and Elizabeth Lopatto, "Lilly Trained Sales Force to Ignore Drug's Risks (Update2)." Bloomberg, July 31, 2008.

   http://www.bloomberg.com/apps/news?pid=newsar- chive&refer=healthcare&sid=a3zg322ZNbDw

7. Elisabeth Rosenthal, "Even Small Medical Advances Can Mean Big Jumps in Bills." *New York Times,* April 5, 2014. http://www.nytimes.com/2014/04/06/health/even-small-medical-advances-can-mean-big-jumps-in-bills.html?partner=rss&emc=rss

8. Brigid Killelea et al., "Evolution of Breast Cancer Screening in the Medicare Population: Clinical and Economic Implications." *Oxford Journal*, May 11, 2014. http://www.oxfordjournals.org/our_journals/jnci/press_releases/killeleadju159.pdf

9. Reed Abelson and Julie Creswell, "Hospital Chain Said to Scheme to Inflate Bills." New York Times, January 23, 2014. http://www.nytimes.com/2014/01/24/business/hospital-chain-said-to-scheme-to-inflate-bills.html?partner=rss&emc=rss&_r=0

10. Scott Shipman and Christine Sinsky, "Expanding Primary Care Capacity By Reducing Waste And Improving The Efficiency Of Care." *Health Affairs*, November, 2013. http://content.healthaffairs.org/content/32/11/1990.abstract?sid=d376c99a-0479-450c-b0e9-713a3e476985

11. Steven Brill, "Bitter Pill: Why Medical Bills Are Killing Us." *TIME*, April 4, 2013. http://time.com/198/bitter-pill-why-medical-bills-are-killing-us/

12. Nerdwallet Health, "Compare knee or hip replacement or reattachment surgery." http://www.nerdwallet.com/health/hospitals

Chapter 6

1. Abraham Verghese, "Treat the Patient, Not the CT Scan." *New York Times,* February 26, 2011. http://www.nytimes.com/2011/02/27/opinion/27verghese.html?pagewanted=2&_r=2&ref=homepage&src=me

2. Gordon Fung et al., "It's Not Too Late: a Dozen Topics Neglected in Medical Training." *San Francisco Medicine*, September, 2013.
http://issuu.com/sfmedsociety/docs/
september_623d6accb9ef00/1?e=3533752/4907839

3. In his classic 1962 book *The Structure of Scientific Revolutions*, Thomas Kuhn explained why it's so difficult to adopt a new view, one that's obviously more useful and elegant than the current one. He recounts the story of Galileo, tried for heresy for his claim that the Earth was not the center of the universe. Galileo died in 1642, and the papal ban on his books wasn't lifted until 1718.

Or take Viennese physician Ignaz Semmelweis, who suggested to his colleagues in the 1880s that fewer delivering mothers might die if their doctors simply washed their hands after performing autopsies. For his pains, Semmelweis was driven out of town and ended his days in a mental hospital. But ten years later, hand washing was mandatory.

Kuhn's point was that our most basic views of the world crystallize into our personal reality. Challenge our sense of reality, you confront our very beings. We'll accept your newfangled idea only when you pry the old one out of our cold, dead fingers.

Chapter 9

1. "Medic" TV series, "White Is the Color."
http://www.youtube.com/watch?v=xErX5vN4s4o

2. Allan Detsky and Harlan Krumholz, "Reducing the Trauma of Hospitalization." *Journal of the American Medical Association*, June 4, 2014.
http://jama.jamanetwork.com/article.aspx?arti-
cleID=1867736&utm_source=Silverchair Information Systems&utm_medium=email&utm_campaign=MASTER:-
JAMALatestIssueTOCNotification06/04/2014

Chapter 11

1. Compassion Fatigue Awareness Project.
   http://www.compassionfatigue.org/

Chapter 13

1. Eliza, Computer Therapist.
   http://www.manifestation.com/neurotoys/eliza.php3

Chapter 14

1. Rachel Aviv, "Prescription for Disaster." *New Yorker*, May 5,
   2014.
   http://www.newyorker.com/magazine/2014/05/05/
   prescription-for-disaster   .

Chapter 15

1. Centers for Disease Control and Prevention, "The Adverse
   Childhood Experiences (ACE) Study."
   http://www.cdc.gov/violenceprevention/acestudy/

Chapter 16

1. "A Controlled Trial to Improve Care for Seriously Ill
   Hospitalized Patients. The Study to Understand Prognoses and
   Preferences for Outcomes and Risks of Treatments.
   (SUPPORT)." *Journal of the American Medical Association*,
   November 22, 1995.
   http://www.ncbi.nlm.nih.gov/pubmed/7474243

Chapter 17

1. Steffie Woolhandler et al, "Is Obamacare Enough? Without
   Single-Payer, Patchwork U.S. Healthcare Leaves Millions
   Uninsured." *Democracy Now*, Oct. 7, 2013.
   http://www.democracynow.org/2013/10/7/
   is_obamacare_enough_without_single_payer

Chapter 18

1. The Lown Institute, "The Right Care Movement."
   http://www.rightcaredeclaration.org/

Chapter 19

1 ISHI, "Remembering the Heart of Medicine"
   http://www.ishiprograms.org/
2. Abby Goodnough, "As Nurse Lay Dying, Offering Herself as
   Instruction in Caring." *New York Times*, January 10, 2013.
   http://www.nytimes.com/2013/01/11/us/fatally-ill-and-mak-
   ing-herself-the-lesson.html?pagewanted=1&_r=2&nl=todays-
   headlines&emc=edit_th_20130111&

Chapter 20

1. For her integrity, Dr. Kelsey was given the President's Award
   for Distinguished Federal Civilian Service in 1962.
   Interestingly, Thalidomide is currently used in the U.S. to
   treat some cancer patients. Since it works by decreasing neo-
   vascularization, it can be disastrous to forming fetal limbs but
   advantageous in depriving tumors of blood supply.

Acknowledgements

1. http://www.amazon.com/Peter-Barnes/e/B001JP9REA/
   ref=sr_tc_2_0?qid=1406577957&sr=1-2-ent

INDEX

S